D0115346

Chicken Soup
for the Soul.

Boost
Your
Brain
Power!

Chicken Soup for the Soul: Boost Your Brain Power!
You Can Improve and Energize Your Brain at Any Age
Dr. Marie Pasinski with Liz Neporent

Published by Chicken Soup for the Soul Health, an imprint of Chicken Soup for the Soul Publishing,
LLC www.chickensoup.com

Front cover and interior photo courtesy of iStockphoto.com/pavlen (© pavlen).
Back cover photo of Dr. Marie Pasinski courtesy of John Mottern.

Cover and Interior Design & Layout by Pneuma Books, LLC
For more info on Pneuma Books, visit www.pneumabooks.com

Distributed to the booktrade by Simon & Schuster. SAN: 200-2442

Publisher's Cataloging-In-Publication Data
(Prepared by The Donohue Group, Inc.)

Pasinski, Marie.

   Chicken soup for the soul : boost your brain power! : you can improve and energize your brain at any
age / Marie Pasinski with Liz Neporent.

   p. ; cm.

   Summary: A collection of stories on the topic of improving brain power, memory, cognitive function,
alertness, accompanied by medical advice.

   ISBN: 978-1-935096-86-3

   1. Brain--Anecdotes. 2. Brain--Care and hygiene--Anecdotes. 3. Brain--Popular works. 4. Brain--Care
and hygiene--Popular works. I. Neporent, Liz. II. Title. III. Title: Boost your brain power

PN6071.B74 P27 2012

810.2/02/356/1   2012931531

PRINTED IN THE UNITED STATES OF AMERICA
on acid∞free paper

21 20 19 18 17 16 15 14 13 12   01 02 03 04 05 06 07 08 09 10

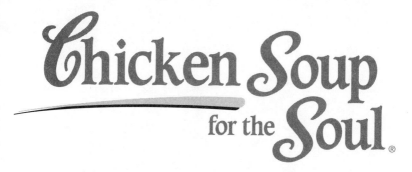

Chicken Soup for the Soul®

Boost Your Brain Power!

You Can Improve and Energize Your Brain at Any Age

by **DR. MARIE PASINSKI** of
HARVARD MEDICAL SCHOOL
with **LIZ NEPORENT**

Chicken Soup for the Soul Publishing, LLC
Cos Cob, CT

Chicken Soup for the Soul

www.chickensoup.com

Contents

Chapter 3

～ **Living Well to Age-Proof the Brain** ～

Chapter 4

～ **Shaping Your Thoughts and Emotions** ～

Chapter 5

～ **Wake Up Your Brain** ～

Chapter 6

～ **Don't Accept Labels** ～

Introduction

"It's the heart."

"It's the brain."

"No, it's the heart!"

"Darling, I KNOW it's the BRAIN!"

My husband and I often have a passionate argument about which organ in the body is the most important. He's an internist and insists it's the heart. If the heart isn't working, he claims, blood doesn't circulate, your cells don't receive oxygen and pretty soon nothing else is working either. As a neurologist, I of course, have no doubt it's the brain. After all, your brain is your very essence—it's what makes you who you are. If your brain isn't functioning, then what's the point? Every once in a while I get him to concede I'm right.

Your brain is a marvel and your most precious possession. Weighing in at just three pounds, it is home to more than one hundred billion neurons interconnected by one hundred trillion synapses, giving rise to your consciousness and your every thought, mood and action. Modern neuroscience research has changed our perception of the brain dramatically. One of the breakthroughs I find most fascinating is our new understanding of the brain's ability to redesign itself. We used to think the brain was static but now recognize that it is incredibly dynamic and constantly evolving. Like a work of art in progress, it's continuously shaped and transformed by experiences and the way it is cared for. No matter your age or your past, it's never too late to take advantage of this remarkable ability.

I can't think of a better way to highlight the potential of the human brain than by pairing stories of innovative individuals creatively using their minds with straightforward scientific explanations of what's taking place in their brains. As the stories so eloquently illustrate, it's possible to change the direction of thoughts, emotions and behaviors, which in turn may transform a moment, a day — or even an entire life. It is thrilling to share with you the explanations of the exciting neuroscience that allows this to happen.

As you read this book, I hope the stories as well as the captivating science inspire you to do more with your brain. Every one of us is capable of reaching our potential. And with no disrespect to the heart or any of the other organs, what better tool to help you get there than your wonderful, amazing brain?

— Marie Pasinski, MD —

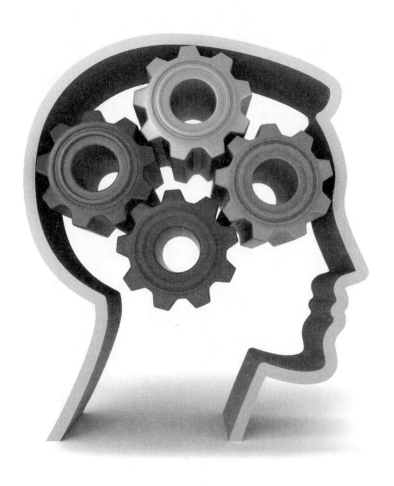

Chapter 1
Invest in
Your Brain

Improving
Through Improv

I stood there like a deer in headlights. "Mom?" Cavin prodded. "Say anything that comes to your mind." All I could think was get me off this stage! Signing up for an improvisational acting class was my son's idea, not mine. He said this class would help me to think quicker and give me the confidence that I needed. I was re-entering the business world after years of being a full-time mom and I made the mistake of complaining to him that I wasn't as sharp as I used to be. I told him how difficult it was for me at a recent networking luncheon to think of things to talk about with the other business people. Instead of giving me the sympathy I was hoping for, Cavin came up with this solution.

Cavin is an actor by profession. When he isn't out of town for film shoots, he teaches acting classes at a Phoenix studio. He is also a favorite performer on various improv stages throughout the valley. Improv is his specialty. It is a form of comedy where the actor must spontaneously create scenes based on the suggestions of the audience. It is a fast-paced performance that leaves the viewer hurting from laughter and marveling over the cleverness that erupts on demand. Cavin told me that improv keeps his mind sharp for auditions and for whatever role he may be called upon to play. Learning this skill would be a great way to help me too. I took the bait.

My first class was abysmal. It started easily enough, with simple exercises to teach us to look our partners directly in the eye and respond to whatever cues they gave us. We played games that challenged our reaction times and exercises that stretched our listening and memory skills. I could see how these exercises would sharpen my brain, and it didn't seem too difficult.

Unfortunately, these were just our warm-up exercises. Cavin then taught us another game called, "Yes, and." We were paired up, and like Noah with his animals, Cavin herded us two by two to center stage. Once stationed in that most intimidating of places, my job was to agree with whatever my partner said about me or the scene and I had to ad lib information to move the scene forward. This was a far more difficult task than our earlier exercises and I found myself tongue-tied or stammering.

"I can't do this," I told Cavin as he drove me home. I was feeling flustered and humiliated. It didn't help that I was the oldest student in the class. My inability to respond quickly like everyone else made me feel older than ever. I expected my son to give me a motivational speech and tell me how I had done better than I thought, but he didn't. Instead he asked, "Why don't you think you can do this?"

"Because I can't think fast enough!" I blurted out in frustration.

"Do you know how you can get better at that?" he calmly asked.

"Yeah," I replied defiantly, "I need to get younger!"

Briefly averting his eyes from the road to glance at me, Cavin smiled and said, "No, by practice."

Now I was angry and frustrated. Tears welled up in my eyes and I looked out the side window at the light poles flying past. What did a 24-year-old know about the way one's thinking slows down as you get older? He didn't understand my fear of getting Alzheimer's disease like my mom did. I silently vowed I would never go back to his improv class. I didn't want to be a comedian anyway.

The following week, when Wednesday rolled around, I tried to put the class out of my mind. Nearly every other night of the week I was parked in a camp chair beside my husband at the baseball field watching Cavin's brother Ryan play college ball. Guilt and my husband prodded me. I needed to give Cavin that one night a week. I swallowed my pride and went back to his improv class.

I liked to watch Cavin teach, and gradually the classes became more fun. I was learning how to quickly invent new characters and scenes, but I still felt terribly inadequate. After each class, Cavin asked me, "How do you think you did?" I told him what I thought worked and what didn't, still unsure of my assessment. But one night I knew I did well!

We were doing a scene that revolved around an imaginary jacket. Dave, the young man on stage, wrapped the jacket around a girl who was pretending to be his girlfriend. She admired the sleeve of the invisible jacket and cooed, "Is that the autograph of the lead singer of the JuJu Bees?"

When Dave drawled, "yea-aah" with a prideful swagger, Cavin yelled, "Show me when he got the autograph!" Immediately, everyone cleared the stage, and like spontaneous combustion I catapulted to the center and mimicked the lead singer of Kiss with abandon! I swung my head, whipping my hair around and around, then stood pumping both fists over my head and stuck out my tongue. I sauntered over to Dave, pulled an imaginary pen from my pocket and scrawled an autograph on the invisible jacket with aplomb.

When I completed that act, I looked around the room and became aware of the eerie silence. Blushing, I resumed my usual demure demeanor and looked back at all the wide, staring eyes. Suddenly, my peers erupted in applause. I had not just stepped out of my comfort zone, I had exploded out of it! Now, I know I won't be stealing any acting jobs from Meryl Streep, but I will say that creative situations came to my mind much faster after that night. I instantly became Queen Elizabeth at a diner, trying to convince the waitress to date my son, or Martha Stewart determined to retouch the paint job on the ceiling of the Sistine Chapel. The improv class became something I looked forward to each week. I was part of the team, contributing to every scene I was in, no longer an anchor dragging it down.

Last week at the dinner table I was bragging to my family that one of the other actors in class told me he preferred to be my partner over everyone else. "He said that I make him better because I am so creative. So, it's working," I gushed, "I'm thinking better! I just wish improv could also improve my math skills."

My college ball player offered, "Mom, you could keep the stats for my team."

"Oh, no," I groaned, "I'd be terrible at that!"

"You know how you get better, don't you?" Cavin calmly asked.

Then grinning, he and Ryan chimed in together, "You practice!"

"I will," I replied. "I'll practice keeping my whining to myself!"

~ Lindy Schneider ~

The Word of the Day

"Hey." I looked up from my computer and my yogurt at the barefoot teenager shuffling into the room.

"Hey," I replied.

Talk radio blared from the counter as she opened the fridge and stared at its contents for a while. She'd been taller than me for a few years, but this year she had gone through a growth spurt, and now she was practically a giant. I watched her grab an apple, tossing it a few times as she carried it to the table. Who was this sporty, confident person who had once been my baby sister?

"So what are we doing today?" she asked.

I took a deep breath and let it out. "I don't know," I said. I really didn't. What did 14-year-olds even do?

Allie and I had been close once, when she was tiny, as in under seven years old. I was in high school at the time, and she would skip into my room, curls bouncing, and sing me the song she learned in kindergarten that day. I would gladly turn away from my chem homework to read to her before bed-time, a chapter of *James and the Giant Peach* or *Anne of Green Gables*, books I'd loved when I was a kid. Over the weeks before I went to college, she cried multiple times at the mere thought of me leaving.

I did go to college, though, and we both adjusted. I made new friends and got invested in my new classes and relationships. When I came home to visit, I focused on catching up with old high school friends. After college, I moved to New York for a job and found love. But each time I returned home, there was more of a distance between Allie and me. Like me, she'd found new friends and activities. She was growing up, and I was too far away to be a part of that experience.

When my partner decided to go back to school, we packed up our New York apartment and prepared for the move to the Midwest town where the college was located. But our move-in date wasn't until late August, and our lease was up July 15th. We decided to spend the month between homes with our respective families. I'd told Allie that it would be a time for us to bond. But now that I was home, I had no idea how we were going to fill the month. I didn't even know her enough to know how she spent her time.

The talk radio program droned on, filling our awkward silence. The novel they were discussing suffered from many growing pains common to the new author. The main character had no agency, and the world in which he lived lacked verisimilitude.

"I always wondered what verisimilitude means," I mused, because at least it was something to say. "I mean, I've heard the word before, but I still have no idea."

"Look it up," said Allie, sounding suspiciously like our mother.

I typed "verisimilitude definition" into Google. "Having the appearance or semblance of truth," I read. Then I looked up at Allie. "Does that make sense?"

"A little," she said. "See if you can find it in a sentence."

I did a little digging, and then read proudly, "In an attempt to create verisimilitude, his dialogue is full of street slang."

I looked at Allie. She grinned at me.

"You know what we should do?" I asked. "We should do this every day. It can be our mission while I'm home to learn a new word each day."

It only sounded incredibly nerdy after I said it out loud. But this was the girl I read *Anne of Green Gables* to as a kid. The apple doesn't fall far from the tree.

"Okay," she said. "But then we have to try and use the words in our normal conversation. Like, just slip them in there."

"We can give each other points for every time we use a word right!" I said.

Thus, The Word of the Day was born.

For the next few mornings, I would bring my laptop to breakfast, and we would spend the first hour of our day eating and looking for words. We laughed a lot, trying to find the funniest-sounding words, coming across the strangest sample sentences, and hearing the best voices when we clicked on pronunciation buttons over and over again. Our favorite word was "agroof," which apparently was an adjective for falling flat on your face. The proper usage? I fell agroof.

Throughout our days, we tried to slip words li
tude" and "blandishment" into our everyday spee
those forced, silly sentences, we learned a lot more ;
other. Allie, I learned, was on the track team at schoo, ..nd her
commitment to running every day, even in the summer when
her coach wasn't checking up on her, was impressive. She was
as disciplined as she was smart.

One day, when I was meeting friends for dinner, she sent
me a text:

"My new contacts added verisimilitude to my run—everything was sharper than usual, so I knew I was indeed in reality."

I was chuckling as I got a second text:

"I expect that you fell agroof in astonishment upon reading
my previous text."

You never know what is going to bring people together.
Sometimes, it's the littlest things—a conversation starter, a
shared challenge, a silly word—that are the most bonding.

When I finally moved, I found myself missing our morning
routine. At least, though, I knew Allie and I had a point of entry
to start our conversation when I called her: What's the word of
the day?

— Eve Legato —

The Gift of Gab

I retired from teaching elementary school six years ago. I enjoyed working with kids, but my body had begun to show the effects of aging—when I'd sit on the floor with the kids, it was harder to get up. And it was more and more tiring to keep up with a group of six-year-olds. So I took advantage of an Early Retirement Incentive, and retired at the ripe old age of 49. With my pension from the state, a part-time job at a local store, and an adjunct position at a local university, I knew I could make ends meet.

My schedule suddenly became a lot more open. I could volunteer with a quilting group at church. I could have lunch with other retirees. I could attend symphony concerts in the middle of the day. I could visit my daughter, who was going to college out of state.

But for some reason, I missed a lot of appointments. How could this happen? When I was the working mom of two active girls, I was able to juggle three schedules and get everyone where they needed to be. It was very frustrating. Even when events were clearly written on my calendar, I either forgot them or arrived late.

One day my cousin came to visit from Japan. He stayed with my parents, and I went to spend some time there. But my cousins don't speak English, and the only person who could speak to him was my mom. She spent much of the time translating. I had taken one Japanese language class in college, but it wasn't nearly enough to carry on a conversation. And then during the hectic child-rearing days, there wasn't enough time to continue learning it.

But now I was a retiree, and had more time. Would it be possible for a middle-aged woman to learn another language? My kids encouraged me to try. By chance, the university where I teach hired a new full-time Japanese professor. I corresponded with him and got permission to audit the class.

On the first day, I nervously showed up with my books and notebook and pencils. I sat in a classroom full of students less than half my age. Even with a lifetime of listening to Japanese and a full year of studying it, I was scrambling to keep up. Learning to read and write Japanese involves not only the extensive vocabulary, but also the hundreds of characters known as kanji. I studied all night for a quiz, only to get a C.

I kept studying. I kept doing the assignments and having Mom check them. Several interesting things happened as I pressed on. I learned compassion for my students who had struggled to read, the ones who couldn't make sense of the marks and swirls we call letters. I learned to have patience for people like my mother, who learned to adapt in a new country, having to understand and speak a new language. And I learned a lot about the culture in which my aunts, uncles, and cousins live.

But the most amazing development was that I started to remember things better. Even though I was busier, going to class and doing the homework, I was better able to keep my appointments, even when Dad passed away suddenly and I had to take care of hundreds of details for Mom. I found myself remembering names and directions. And I became more efficient with my time.

I'm not sure if I'm happier when I'm busy, or if the busyness forces me to plan my day better, but having this extra endeavor has really been a wonderful adventure for me. Last summer, after two years of study, I went to Japan with my mom and my daughter and son-in-law. I still can't carry on much of a conversation with my relatives, and I still can't read enough of the street signs to get around, but it was so much more enjoyable than my previous trip there 25 years earlier.

Last fall I attended the third-year language class with renewed enthusiasm. I began to correspond with my cousins by e-mail, using my poor grammar and limited vocabulary. I always knew I had cousins overseas, but I now have a closer relationship with them. Another bonus!

I got my game back. Life is good.

— Patricia Gordon —

Ready? Set. Go!

I f you want to kick your brain into overdrive, give it a little competition!

A few years back, I'd slipped into a writing rut. I was writing mostly full-time then. But I'd fallen into a few bad habits. I spent hours writing blog posts, or updating on a social network, or reading about writing. Basically, I was in front of my laptop the entire day, but I wasn't really producing anything creative. My imagination seemed to have dried up.

It just so happened that my dry spell came along about the same time as an annual poem-a-day competition. It's a simple concept. For the month of April, we were challenged to write a poem based on a prompt. It didn't have to be pages long; it could be a haiku. But in order to "win," competitors had to produce a poem every single day in April.

Honestly, I'm more of a fiction and essay writer. But I love poetry. Especially short poems. So I took the challenge, knowing that a competition would bring out my primordial need to win, to push myself over the finish line. Plus, maybe I'd jumpstart better writing habits.

It's not that I wanted to write a poem a day for the rest of my life. And I didn't expect much, as far as the poetry went. But I desperately wanted to prod those brain cells out of their safe little box and into wild, open and creative spaces.

At first, it was difficult. Who am I kidding? It was very

difficult! I wanted to put off that prompt like I was a five-year-old running from her mom and the spoonful of medicine! But after the first few days of waiting till the last minute to get the creative juices flowing, I sat myself down and gave myself a good talking-to. I decided that I would write the poem first thing in the morning. Or at least check out the prompt so I could think about it during the day.

By Day 7, I'd started my new routine. I'd check the prompt in mid-morning when it was posted. Then I'd go about mundane writing chores, take a shower, eat lunch, and maybe run an errand. By the time I sat down to write again, my brain had been mulling over that prompt for a couple of hours.

Sometimes, it took all day to think up a few brilliant lines. But by the end of the evening, I always got my poem finished. By the end of the month, I had 30 poems. I'd "won" the competition! And here's what I'd won:

I won bragging rights to say I wrote a poem a day for the month of April.

I won a few poetry contests when I later took some of my favorite poems, polished them up, and sent them off for competitions.

I won a little confidence, feeling that I could, in fact, write a pretty decent poem.

Mostly, though, I pushed myself out of that writing rut and produced every single day. I exercised my creativity and imagination, and limbered up my problem-solving skills. (Don't believe me? Try writing a villanelle.) I learned something new about poetry almost every single day. I felt like my brain exploded in April—in a good way, of course.

Now, when I feel a rut coming on, I find another writing-every-day competition. I've done National Novel Writing Month, and I give myself serious daily writing goals, too. But I have to admit that public competitions work better for me. I suppose it's a little bit of pride. Once I've put myself out there and signed up, I have to cross that finish line.

Why not try a write-every-day competition and see where your brain takes you? No one has to see the results except you. But don't be surprised when glorious and creative thoughts cross the finish line!

— Cathy C. Hall —

Invest in Your Brain

Introduction

In my tiny community, there is a coffee shop at the edge of town where I often stop on my way to work. Every morning a group of older men gather there to do the New York Times crossword puzzle together. I love listening to the steady buzz of social energy that fills the shop as they work their puzzles, chat, laugh and toss out clues to one another. Naturally, as a neurologist, I can't help but admire how much good these men are doing for their brains.

There are the puzzles of course. These help the men flex their memories and challenge their verbal skills. But since they've been doing the crossword for years, they may have maxed out the learning potential of this particular task. What's doing their brains the most good is the fact that they get together, interact and engage in a lively exchange of ideas. Thinking about the answers to their puzzle may be a stimulating intellectual exercise in its own right, but the social experience of doing the puzzles together, sharing ideas and engaging in lively conversation is what makes their gatherings a true brain boosting activity.

Enrich Your Mind

High quality social connections appear to protect against

cognitive decline. Recent studies show a 25 percent reduction in the risk of developing dementia among seniors who report feeling satisfied with the relationships in their lives. Having an interesting and fulfilling social life into your golden years is just one of several factors that may help preserve the brain's store of knowledge and memory, a concept known as cognitive reserve.

A robust cognitive reserve is essential for keeping your mind sharp as you age. One recent study reported that nearly 40 percent of people who die without any measurable cognitive deficits have evidence of Alzheimer's disease in their brains. These include the hallmark plaques and tangles.

How can this be? We now understand that some people seem to tolerate the pathologic brain changes of Alzheimer's pretty well. It appears that having a well-funded intellectual savings account somehow compensates for whatever damage has accumulated in the brain. When there's a pile-up or traffic jam on your main neural highways, cognitive reserve serves as an alternate route for information to travel. So, even if your preferred cognitive route is blocked, you still have a side exit and smaller streets available to get you to your destination. True, it may take you longer to get there, but at least you won't be stuck indefinitely.

Scientists didn't always believe there were ways to build up cognitive reserve throughout an entire lifetime. They used to think the brain behaved like cement: Young, freshly poured neural pathways could swiftly absorb materials and impressions but eventually these pathways would become set in stone, hardened and intractable with age. We now know this is far from true: The brain is more like a glorious garden, capable of growing, blooming and sending out new roots when the conditions are favorable. Research has shown that stimulating experiences and new learning, like sunshine and rain, allow this garden to flourish—and that's true whether you are young or old.

The Miracle of Neuroplasticity

Regardless of age, your brain has the ability to make new neurons and construct new neural pathways throughout your life. Every time you engage in new activities, think in novel ways, learn a skill or do things differently, new pathways are forged and your cognitive reserve expands. This process, called neuroplasticity, has been a revelation in neuroscience.

Numerous studies have helped us to understand how learning transforms the brain. Take, for example, a landmark German study of a group of people who had never juggled before. After giving them three months of juggling training, the investigators scanned the newly minted jugglers' brains and found an increase in volume of areas that process complex visual motion. Although the change was temporary, the study demonstrated an anatomical modification as a result of learning.

Another study by German researchers looked at the effect of intense studying on brain structure. Medical students preparing for their board exams underwent MRI scans of their brains before, during and three months after they completed their exams. The students experienced a significant volume increase in various brain regions including the hippocampus (the brain's memory center) over time. And what's even more exciting is that three months after they stopped studying for exams, the student's hippocampi continued to enlarge. This is thought to be due to the proliferation of new neurons induced by learning.

Every part of the brain serves a special function. In recent years, there's been an explosion of research in the field of neuroplasticity. Using MRI technology, the brains of athletes, musicians, video gamers and even cabdrivers have been studied. This has provided a new understanding of how the brain is shaped by the way it's utilized. For example, the scan of an accomplished pianist will show expansion of the cortical areas associated with finger dexterity while those of experienced cabdrivers reveal enlargement of regions dedicated to spatial navigational skills.

Researchers have even begun looking at how brain structure may be molded by online social networks. They've found that college students with more friends on Facebook had enlargement of various brain regions, including an area linked with the task of putting names to faces. For me, this kind of research underscores the fact that the brain you have at this very moment mirrors the way you have spent your time. But more importantly, the future structure of your brain is yet to be determined.

Making Friends for Your Brain's Sake

I've already mentioned that having lots of friends is associated with maintaining mental performance and increasing cognitive reserve. My older acquaintances from the coffee shop, with their vibrant social lives, are a good example of this. And this is true even after other factors such as whether a person suffers from depression or other illnesses have been accounted for. There's something about being social that's good for the brain. What might this be?

Think about the possibilities a social encounter presents. Say, for example, you bump into a friend while you're out grocery shopping. You get to talking about the old neighborhood, which you haven't thought about in years, and then she invites you to a new play that's just opened at the local theater. The next night you attend the play, where she introduces you to a new group of friends. You find yourself immersed in the ideas presented in the play and by your new acquaintances. Afterwards you and the group go out to a Moroccan restaurant that you've never been to before. At dinner someone invites you to join her tennis group. You accept enthusiastically and over the next few weeks this inspires you to get in shape. Plus you meet another new set of people at the tennis club. And so on... One simple conversation in the cereal aisle leads to an interwoven tapestry of experiences you never would have had sitting home alone in front of the TV.

Whereas passive activities like TV watching put your brain into neutral gear, social interaction shifts it into high gear, calling upon it to perform a variety of complex tasks including those that require memory, attention, reasoning and language skills. Your brain is stimulated in countless ways that seem to energize the brain for other intellectual functions as well—this in turn expands your cognitive reserve.

We also know that having friends to lean on in times of strife helps you weather life's stormier events. Stressful emotions such as anxiety, depression and loneliness take their toll on the brain. The emotional support provided by close personal relationships seems to cushion some of those cognitive blows. They can also help you reframe problems in a more positive way and discover new solutions. Two brains are always better than one!

The More You Know, the More You Know

Do you remember what life was like when you were young? For most of us, every day was an adventure. There was always something new going on. You were continually challenged, learning and discovering. Your brain was busy contemplating new concepts, developing new skills and adding to your cognitive reserve. But then you graduated from school. Over the years you gradually settled into a standard routine with work, family and friends, repeating many of the same kinds of tasks and activities over and over. You didn't stop gathering new information altogether—but you didn't gather it at anywhere near the pace of your youth.

During the early developmental stages of your life, you formed millions of neural connections. Some ultimately are pruned away, but those that survived connected with other neurons during the rapid-growth stage of the nervous system that occurred in childhood and adolescence. Reading progressively more challenging books, developing new talents, creating art, playing games, meeting people, going new places—engaging in a variety of mentally stimulating activities — helped form these vital neural connections that folded into your cognitive reserve.

My question to you is this: Why stop there? There's no physiological reason that the deliberate funding of your cognitive reserve should cease the moment you're handed your last diploma. If you continue to challenge your mind, embrace new activities and acquire new skills you can continue to build up neural connections indefinitely.

One proven way to do this is indeed to pursue as much education and as many diplomas as possible. Studies show that the more time you've spent hitting the books, the lower the risk of Alzheimer's. The same conclusions have been drawn about those who work at highly complex, intellectually demanding jobs.

But not to worry if you didn't get a Ph.D. Formal education is only one way to stimulate the brain. I have, for example, an 84-year-old neighbor who is the perfect role model for how to maintain a healthy, vibrant brain as you age. Every time I talk to her she always has some fascinating new experience to share with me. She's either just returning from a biking trip in France or taking a class in furniture refinishing or reading the most interesting book. On her eightieth birthday she jumped off the local pier into the ocean with her children and grandchildren! In many ways she lives her life like a perpetual college student, filling her time and mind with a steady stream of new and novel experiences and ideas. And believe me when I tell you, she's as mentally sharp as they come.

Boosting Your Brain Power

I wish everyone would seize the day like my neighbor does once their school days are behind them. As we get older, many of us fall into an intellectual rut. The construction of new neural circuits is put on hold as the demand for new ways of thinking dwindles. When I lecture, I often ask attendees if they've taken up a new hobby in the past year. Usually only a few hands go up. What about the past two, three or even five years, I ask them next. Even then, a minority raise their hands. We know that life-long learning lowers your risk of dementia. So if you truly want to build your cognitive reserves, it's time to start challenging your mind.

It begins by opening yourself up to new experiences. In our everyday life there are countless opportunities that can stimulate new ways of thinking. It could be as simple as attending a lecture on a topic that interests you, playing a new game or listening to a new genre of music. Like the cereal aisle vignette above, small changes in our routine have a way of snowballing.

Instead of going to the movies this weekend, why not go dancing? Many clubs now offer free lessons at the beginning of the evening. Or, like Cathy Hall described in the story "Ready? Set. Go!", why not write a poem a day for a month to get your creative juices flowing? Engaging in new activities that are physical and social further boosts the brain benefits, as they also deliver the neuroprotective effects of exercise and socialization.

I encourage you to commit to trying something new every week. Engaging in new experiences on a regular basis will ultimately make learning a way of life. Keep a journal to track your progress. This will not only reinforce what you have learned, but it will also instill learning as a lifelong habit. When learning becomes a habit you will constantly be transforming and updating the infrastructure of your brain.

When you're ready, think bigger. To fully reap the benefits of neuroplasticity, a deeper commitment is required. Immersing yourself in a challenging pursuit is the best way to endow your cognitive reserve. It doesn't take learning rocket science or for that matter, brain science, to shift neuroplasticity into high gear. In fact, choosing any endeavor that you are passionate about will enhance the learning process.

For example, if you've always been fascinated with Spanish or Latino culture, why not learn how to speak the language? Take a leap, as Patricia Gordon did in her story "The Gift of Gab," and sign up for a class. If you're an independent learner, try a software program or listen to instructional audiotapes. Practice your skills by watching movies in Spanish with subtitles, singing along with Marc Anthony, dining at authentic restaurants or preparing a Latino feast (using a cookbook written in Spanish of course!) Making friends with native speakers or traveling to destinations where Spanish is spoken are fun ways to further develop your burgeoning skills.

The possibilities to expand your intellectual horizons are endless. Whether you learn to play a musical instrument, take a computer class or dedicate yourself to the art and sport of horseback riding, have fun with it. All of these are wonderful examples of complex activities that require multiple cognitive skills and challenge your brain to think and grow in new directions.

No matter when you start or how much you've done until now, you can endlessly deposit more knowledge and experience into the coffers of your cognitive reserve.

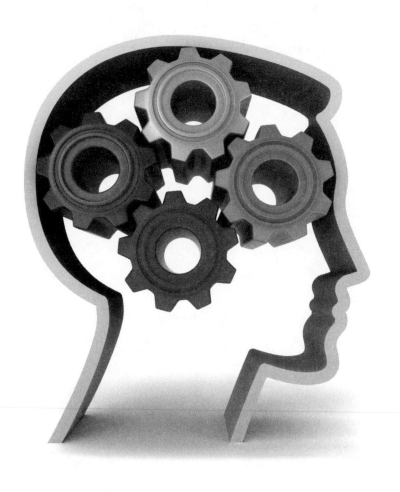

Chapter 2
Your Amazing Memory

Capital of Delaware

"**M**om, can you help me out? What's the capital of Delaware?" My eight-year-old son, Samuel, looked up from his paper with wide, green eyes.

"I'm not going to tell you, Mister Man," I said. "Look it up."

"I'll see if I can remember," Samuel said. Then he rattled off most of the states in the East, capitals and all, but Delaware he couldn't recall.

"C'mon, Mom," he said. "I know you know."

"Look it up," I said with a smile. "I'll hand you the map."

I offered Samuel a small U.S. map, brightly colored states protected with shiny laminate. It was best for Samuel to find his own capital, but the truth was, I couldn't recall the city if I tried. Even though we'd been studying the 50 states and their capitals for our home school geography, the capital of Delaware, and most of the others, escaped me.

It just wasn't there.

"Dover," Samuel said, smile wide and wonderful, his finger pressed against the map.

"Awesome," I said. But I was still troubled that I couldn't remember what I'd learned just the day before.

The Dover incident wasn't an isolated occurrence, and that

bothered me. Maybe it was because my husband and I had five children and our home was filled with people coming and going, busyness, and constant stimulation. Maybe it was just a matter of too much going on. System overload. My brain couldn't collect all the information that rushed in. Some information was bound to spill out. Like state capitals.

I believed this for a while. It seemed feasible. Too much input. But then one afternoon, I got a phone call from the orthodontist's office. Apparently someone had forgotten my son Grant's checkup. We'd have to reschedule. But it would take three weeks.

"I feel terrible that Grant's appointment is so far out," I said to my husband, later that evening. "I can't believe I forgot to take him to get his braces checked."

"Everyone drops the ball once in a while," he said.

"Plus I couldn't remember the capital of Delaware."

"What? Shawnelle, Grant's teeth will be fine. It's all okay."

But in my heart, it wasn't. This constant inability to remember things was getting me down.

The next day, my sons and I gathered in our home school classroom. It was Friday, and many of our tests were saved for the end of the week. Samuel had a science test. I paged through his fourth grade test booklet, skimming the essay questions. We'd been studying forces and machines. But as I read through the questions, I was challenged. What was the definition for force? How does a block and tackle decrease the effort needed to do work?

Could I answer these questions, not in general, but according to the text, material I'd covered the week before?

I wasn't sure. But it seemed like a challenge. I copied Samuel's test page, and resolved to see what my brain had retained.

"What are you doing, Mom?" Samuel asked, when I pulled my chair next to his and slid a test in front of each of us.

"Taking your test," I said.

Then I sat down and scribbled like mad, taking the test, right next to my son.

The result furthered my conviction to remember more, to do better.

This gnawed at my brain, the next day, while I went for my morning run. My feet hit the pavement with a steady rhythm. Thud thud. Thud thud. Why was retaining information such a problem? Then an idea began to percolate in my mind. Though the result was frustrating, maybe I was on the right track, taking that science test. Maybe my brain needed to be stretched and exercised, just like my body. The brain is a muscle, too. Keeping my legs fit and strong was an ongoing challenge, especially since I'd hit the big four-O. It made good sense that the same would be true of my brain.

A mental workout was just what I needed. I sprinted the rest of the way home, excited to share my new plan.

The opportunities for cognitive exercise were endless. Possibilities lurked around every corner. When the kids and I went shopping, I'd spend a few minutes looking at the list, and then Samuel would quiz me as I drove to the store. On Bible club night, after the kids had nailed their memory verses, I'd re-cite the same verses, too. We memorized poetry during lunch. And then there were the science and history tests. I took every one. I wondered if my brain was becoming more fit with this exercise, just like the muscles in my legs and arms. Then one day the boys and I watched a nature show on television. My little sons were drawn in by the details of the koala. They were so excited. After the documentary, we found an article online.

When Lonny got home for dinner, the boys were a fount of information.

"Dad, koalas aren't bears at all," Samuel said, over his plate of spaghetti and sauce.

"Really? Please pass the salad," Lonny said. "Where do they live?"

"Australia," another little son piped.

"So why aren't they bears?"

I speared a green leaf with my fork. "English-speaking set-tlers in the 18th century thought that they were bears, because they resembled bears. But Samuel's right. They're not bears. They're marsupials." I munched my salad and recalled a few more cool facts. "And do you know, they eat only eucalyptus leaves, which are poisonous to anything other than the koala. They have a special digestive system that enables them to eat the plants."

"Really?" Lonny asked.

Our little boys nodded.

"Yeah," I said. "And they have special storage in their mouths, too. To save food for later." I thought for a minute. "The female can have a baby once a year for about 12 years."

Lonny beamed over the table. "Listen to you. Seems that your mental workouts are working."

I smiled at his observation. I guess they were! Gentle gladness filled my heart. Not in a haughty, proud way, but with a quiet, accomplished sort of pleasure. Like when I ran my first mile.

"I think you're right," I said.

Lonny winked.

"And the capital of Delaware," I added, as I speared some more lettuce, "is Dover."

~ Shawnelle Eliasen ~

Picking My
Brain Booster

I've been absentminded since birth. As a kid I was forever losing things—combs, watches, baseball gloves—you name it. My hands had the ability to operate independently of any cerebral process, as if they had a mind of their own.

My mind would center on something of interest while, unbeknownst to it, my hand would put whatever it was holding in a spot where it would never be found again. I understand why my Irish ancestors believed in those prankish wee folk—leprechauns and fairies—who sneak around and hide things.

No doubt, if I were in the third grade today, I would be force-fed Ritalin or some such pharmaceutical. But my third grade experience was at a two-room country school, and the only substance that was abused was leather—the teacher's belt used bullwhip-style—which even experienced vicariously was an effective behavior modification modality.

Modern prescriptions may work, but I'm not interested. Nor am I interested in any focus-rendering supplements (clinically shown to improve memory in rats), ginkgo biloba, or other nostrums sold in health food stores.

Age has not improved my absentmindedness. If anything, it has compounded the problem with age-related issues such as short-term memory impairment, "senior moments," and CRS (Can't Remember Stuff).

So after countless incidents of staring vacantly into the refrigerator because I couldn't remember why I had opened it, or going on scavenger hunts several times a week because I couldn't find my car keys, I decided to take action before I was placed in a nursing home before my time.

Articles abound in popular magazines and on the Internet about the importance of exercising the senior mind to stay vital and engaged. The mind is like a muscle they say—use it or lose it. My wife's solution is Sudoku, that mind-boggling numbers grid invented by an ingenious Swiss fellow in 1793 and popularized more recently by a Japanese publisher. But that's too much like arithmetic for someone who got a "C" in college algebra.

My 80-something mother-in-law, whose mind in many ways is more capable than mine, has worked crossword puzzles all her life. Crossword puzzles are not for me. They involve too many arcane words like "ova" and esoteric names of Greek muses or the moons of Jupiter.

Then there's the old standard—learn a new language. Not for me, either. That would mean going to class at night. I spent seven years teaching evening classes at a community college, and I'm too old for that, now. And, as my wife will attest, my brain shuts down after 8:00 p.m.

Recently, I heard that learning to play a musical instrument was good for the developing brains of children, as well as the declining minds of seniors. Some experts say that playing an instrument is even better than doing crossword puzzles! Now, there was a possibility; it sounded better than sitting in front of the county courthouse whittling with the other codgers.

The piano was out of the question—entirely too intimidating. But what about a banjo? Who wouldn't like to be able to play a banjo? A banjo looked like it would be fun and has a certain amount of cachet. How hard could it be? I'd seen hillbillies on *Hee Haw* make it look easy. Even a comedian like Steve Martin learned to play a five-string banjo. I didn't expect to be a virtuoso such as Earl Scruggs—just five easy pieces was all I needed.

Since I had plinked a guitar for years and had most campfire songs and a few Beatles tunes in my repertoire, I thought I'd have a running start with a banjo.

Then my aging mind, which still tries to engage in fancy footwork and look for loopholes, decided that learning new chords for the banjo would be an unnecessary, tedious process. An intermediate step might be the solution. A banjitar.

A banjitar is a hybrid instrument that looks like a banjo but has six strings like a guitar. It is designed to sound like a banjo but is fingered like a guitar. To my mind, it would be the best of both worlds, with no pesky new chords to learn. My mind justified the thought by reminding me that the Old Crow Medicine Show, a popular string band, employs a banjitar.

My mind was doing the Texas two-step, now. It still had CRS, but it was on a roll: Buy a banjitar on eBay. One hundred dollars and a few days later, the banjitar arrived. It fell short of my expectations. The sound it produced was like a fork on a pan.

Asking for help is always the last refuge for me. I called a music store in the city and told an instructor about my banjitar. He said he provided instruction in bluegrass-style picking, which would not work on a six-string banjitar. He added that I could rent a five-string banjo if I wanted to take lessons. I signed up for four Saturday sessions.

At my first lesson, I advised the instructor that I just needed to learn five easy pieces, but in no time at all, I was convinced there weren't five easy pieces. Not on the banjo. Not even "Turkey in the Straw" or "The Ballad of Jed Clampett."

With a five-string banjo, the lower four strings extend from the bottom all the way to the top of the neck. The top string only goes about halfway up the neck and produces a high-pitched tone that is integral to the bluegrass sound.

With four strings on the upper neck and five on the bottom, my mind believes, and sabotages my hands into believing, that when my left hand is playing the top string on the neck that my right hand should be playing the top string on the bottom. Wrong. The top string on the bottom is the fifth (short) string. The result is a piercing whine that sounds like a bullet ricocheting off a church bell.

For the accomplished picker, the banjo is truly a musical instrument. For me, it is a neuro-motor skills appliance that challenges both hemispheres of my brain. On the neck of the banjo, the right brain controls the fingers of the left hand to make individual notes and chords. On the strumming part, the left brain manipulates curled fingers in continuous rolling patterns. But getting the left hand and the right hand to work independently is like patting your head and rubbing your belly at the same time. It can be done, but only with serious practice.

It's been a year since I started lessons. Have my memory and mental faculties improved? As Mao Tse-tung supposedly said in remarking on the effect of the French Revolution—it's too soon to tell. But nonetheless, there are collateral benefits. I no longer fret about avoiding Sudoku and crossword puzzles, and I experience a lofty, insufferable smugness when a stranger sees my banjo case and wistfully says, "I always wanted to play the banjo."

Smugness is a precarious perch. A few weeks ago, as I was getting in my car after a lesson, my instructor hustled out of his studio waving some papers to get my attention. "Hey, professor, you forgot your music."

Maybe I should give up and join the geezers at the courthouse after all.

— L.D. Whitaker —

B My Hero

"Will you water the garden?" my husband asks, putting on his suit jacket.

I rub sleep from my eyes. "Yeah."

I'm not even out of bed yet, and already I feel bad. Before my husband planted a garden I agreed to water it. He reminds me every morning, though most days I forget and he does it when he gets home.

"Could you remember to get my shirts from the cleaner today? If you don't think you can do it, tell me, and I'll pick them up on my way home."

He doesn't sound mad, but I get the impression he's disappointed in me. He asked twice last week and I forgot both times.

"I'll do it." My voice is terse. I'm not mad at him; I'm mad at me. The minute the garage door closes I get a tube of lipstick and draw a red C on the mirror above my sink. When I see it later in the day, it'll remind me to go to the cleaner. I add a G for garden and crawl back in bed. I don't have to get up for another 20 minutes. Maybe if I sleep until then, I won't feel so exhausted.

But I don't sleep. I stare at the ceiling. After the school bus leaves, I drag my slippered feet to the kitchen sink and rinse cereal bowls. The dishwasher needs unloading. It might as well be a truckload of frozen salmon I have to debone. I can't even contemplate doing it until I've rested. I glance into the living room where the couch glows like a neon sign, beckoning me. What's wrong with me? How did I ever teach all day? I feel so ashamed.

Even if I had the energy to teach again, I'd never be able to hide my dimwittedness at work. At home I can mask my brain's deterioration in repeated menial tasks. Dishes, laundry, floors. Dishes, laundry, floors. But at work, I'd be found out. I'd make mistakes and look stupid and people would see that the cheese had long slipped off my cracker. I might return one day from recess with my kindergarten brood only to discover I'd for-gotten Billy-the-Hider on the playground. The principal would enter my classroom, her fist clasping the scruff of Billy's collar, glaring at me over the top of her glasses. "Forget something?" she'd say, and my dirty little secret would be out.

Maybe if I sit down and take care of the phone calls, the dishwasher won't seem so daunting when I get back up. Last night I made a list of the calls I have to make, in case I couldn't remember them today. Now, if I could just remember where I put that list. I slog from room to room, searching. The kids have gotten toothpaste all over the bathroom sink. I turn on the faucet and shuffle into the kitchen to get the bottle of Pine-Sol. On the closet door, where I keep the cleaning supplies, is the Post-it note listing the calls I want to make. I grab it and take a seat at the desk, next to the phone. The first call I make is to the dentist. I apologize for missing my appointment yesterday and schedule another. I call Aetna next to request claims forms for a recent surgery.

"Sure, we can send that," the agent says. "Give me your address."

I open my mouth and am suddenly aware that I don't remember my own address. My heart pounds; my palms grow sweaty with fear. I hang up the phone before the agent suspects a botched lobotomy. I sink to the floor and cry. I'm too young. I have kids to raise. My head drops to my knees and I close my eyes. There, on the inside of my lids, I see it. 429 North Fifth Street. Too late.

I decide to schedule an appointment with my family doctor.

Sitting in her office, I confess my shameful, rapid aging. Six months ago I told her about the mood swings and fatigue. She put me on antidepressants, but they just aren't doing the trick. This time I disclose my memory loss.

The doctor explains that there are many things that can cause memory problems. Most people who are having memory problems automatically fear they are at the early stages of dementia or Alzheimer's disease, but in fact there are many medical conditions that can impact brain functioning. The doctor is mindful of my recent chemo and radiation treatments, runs some tests and finds I have a vitamin B-12 deficiency. I start taking B-12 injections.

By the end of the month, the mental fog is lifted—my thoughts, clear and sunny. I notice a huge improvement in my memory and stamina. I am ready to take on the day with energy and enthusiasm. I go out to water the garden, lipstick G's no longer required, and when I return I nudge my husband, who's asleep in bed. "Wake up, honey. Remember, you have a dentist appointment before work today."

I still occasionally forget things, (where I left my keys, for example) but I never forget to thank God each and every day that my doctor knew to check my B-12 level. I don't know if I would have even told the doctor about my memory problems if it hadn't been for my cancer treatment, but I am glad that I did, and I recommend that everyone tell their doctor if they start to notice memory problems.

~ Kim Hackett ~

Partly Cloudy Pancakes

I t wasn't until eleventh grade that anyone told me how to take notes.

Teachers always told me that I needed to take notes. That I needed to review my notes. That I needed to study my notes before exams. But nobody ever told me how to take notes, not until eleventh grade.

My history teacher, Mr. Provencher, was a leprechaun of a man—short, always smiling, slightly disheveled. He was sprightly, sometimes hopping from foot to foot.

He also clapped when he changed subjects, as if to wake those of us sitting in the back row.

Clap, clap. "Notes. You're going to want to take lots of notes in this class. I'm going to be doing a lot of talking and a lot of your grade is going to be dependent on how well you repeat what I've said."

He paced the first row, grinning all the while. "But I talk fast. Unless you're a natural born stenographer, you're not going to be able to capture every word I utter. So what words do you scribble down in your notebooks?

"Dates, of course. This is a history class. The names of people and places and battles. The names of treaties, doctrines, and pacts. Movements, amendments, and laws.

"But what do they mean? A date without context is meaningless. Do you even know what context means? Should you write it down?"

Again he clapped. "Let's forget about history for a moment. As if you could. As if every fact you've ever heard isn't already stored in your brain."

He tapped the side of his head. "Your brain records every word I say. Every word said by every teacher you've ever had. So why don't you ace every exam?"

Mr. Provencher walked to the blackboard, picked up a piece of chalk, and proceeded to bang out a sky's worth of stars.

Tap, tap, tap, tap, tap.

He turned to face us. "There it is, a map of all you've ever heard. And yet, come the day of the pop quiz, you stare at the blank space and you can't remember the causes of the French and Indian War."

Mr. Provencher reached behind and circled one of the dots. "The answer's right there. You just couldn't find it. Why? Because facts all look alike."

After putting down the chalk, Mr. Provencher blew the dust from his fingers.

"So. The day of the big exam. How do you find that fact hidden among all the others in your brain? Raise your hand if you have any suggestions for your fellow students."

"Study."

"Studying helps, yes. Next?" Mr. Provencher pointed to someone else from the first row.

"Memorize the textbook."

Mr. Provencher nodded. "Doing the assigned reading helps, yes. And just because I assign chapter one tonight doesn't mean you can't read it again later in the semester. Someone from the back?"

"Look at someone else's paper."

Snickers and high fives failed to knock Mr. Provencher off his stride.

"That's right. And do you know why looking at someone else's paper works? Context. Context allows you to give meaning to dry facts. The more context you add, the easier it is for you to find something. Which brings us back to taking notes."

Mr. Provencher clapped. "If you just write facts in your notebook, you'll have a collection of facts. They're already in your brain. Yes, writing them down helps you remember them, but to really make them useful, add context. I'm going to tell you how."

Mr. Provencher sat on the edge of his desk. "Every class, before you start taking notes, write the date." He pointed at the window. "Describe the weather. Put down what you ate for breakfast, or what you said to your parents that morning, or something that happened on the ride in. Draw a face that reflects your mood."

He hopped up from the desk. "When you make these personal notes, you add context to the facts you're going to scribble down, and this makes it easier for you to recall them when you're looking at that pop quiz or exam.

"Everybody that doesn't have their notebook already open

should open their notebook. Write the date, and then jot down some of the other personal items I mentioned. When you're ready, we'll begin."

The causes of the French and Indian War?

That's the day it was supposed to be sunny, but clouds piled up while I waited for the bus, the day I had pancakes for breakfast. Causes of the French and Indian War?

I remember them still.

~ Stephen D. Rogers ~

Your Amazing Memory

Introduction

When I waited tables during my high school and college years, I used to practice the waitress equivalent of flying on a trapeze without a safety net—I wouldn't jot down any of the orders I took. Instead, I would keep my pad in my pocket, concentrate on what my customers requested and memorize everything. Sure, I'd make the occasional mistake on a table of 10 or on some particularly complicated substitution. But you'd be surprised at how few errors I made, especially once I'd been doing it for a while.

This little exercise was great training for later in life. My keen memory gave me an edge during medical school and now as a busy neurologist it helps me still. But understand, it's not as if I was born some sort of memory superstar. Like any other skill, training and good technique are key. Anyone with a normally functioning brain can sharpen memory. With practice, dedication and some strategy, improved memory is one of those capabilities that are within reach of the average person.

How Memory Works

Having a good memory is not the same thing as having perfect teeth, nice eyes or great hair. Memory doesn't exist in the same way body parts do. When neurologists speak of memory they refer to the act of remembering, a process that's spread throughout various areas of the brain as opposed to being concentrated in one single location. And rather than something that happens all at once, memory is a fluid, multifaceted and ongoing brain activity. Let me explain what I mean by that.

Whenever I evaluate a patient's memory I ask them to repeat and remember these three words: ball, tree, shoe. Asking the patient to repeat the three words evaluates what we refer to in neurology as "immediate recall." I distract them briefly by asking a couple of unrelated questions, and then ask them to repeat the three items again, testing short-term memory.

Memory formation is a sequential operation where information processing moves from the present (immediate recall) into short-term memory and then into long-term memory. This exercise tests immediate recall and short-term memory. In order to remember something it first has to appear on your radar screen. If it doesn't, it never registered and it can't possibly be remembered. Someone with significant memory or attentional difficulties will be unable to repeat the words immediately after I say them, while someone who can't recall these words a few minutes later may have short-term memory issues.

Every day your short-term memory is filled with new facts, names, events, concepts and impressions. Most of these short-term memories are not that important and decay over time. For example, I don't expect my patients to remember the three words I gave them when they come for their follow up visit several weeks later; this information isn't important enough to store in their long-term memory. Besides, I can easily test their long-term memory by asking them to name the last three presidents of the United States or what happened on September 11, 2001.

So how does the brain retain memories? Information streams into your brain through the five senses (sight, sound, smell, taste and touch.) When I say sensory information streams what I'm really describing is a flood. You couldn't possibly attend to every bit of data that comes at you from the outside world, so your brain is forced to prioritize.

Immediate recall has a small storage capacity. Experts have determined it can only hold about seven independent items at one time. This is one of the reasons information like local phone numbers and zip codes are seven digits or less. It's too difficult to hold longer strings of numbers in your head for the amount of time it takes to press the buttons on your phone or write on an envelope. It's also why breaking up numbers like phone numbers and social security numbers into separate and distinct chunks of data makes them easier to remember.

Information from immediate recall is only sent into short-term memory under certain circumstances. Unless you purposefully make an effort to remember something, you'll only retain a memory if it's an attention grabber — like a parade of clowns marching up Main Street — something that's emotionally meaningful — picking up a loved one at the train station — or any piece of intel that is personally important to you — for example, a job interview is much less likely to slip your mind than a routine dental cleaning.

Memories become permanent keepsakes and enter long-term memory when they are truly learned, emotionally significant, personally meaningful or especially memorable. The brain attaches newer memories to similar and related memories to enable you to consolidate new concepts and facts with older memories. However, just because something has been stored in your memory, doesn't mean you can necessarily access it immediately.

We've all experienced "tip of the tongue syndrome," that maddening memory malfunction where you try to call up some word, name or fact and you can almost see the information but can't quite grab it from your memory bank. In effect, you remember that you remember something — though you can't actually remember what it is you're trying to remember! This is a problem with retrieval — the process that allows you to bring stored memories into conscious awareness when needed. Because similar information is often stored together, cues can be helpful in triggering that elusive word or memory.

Memory Hitches and Glitches

Those little memory lapses we're all prone to, like misplacing keys and forgetting names, can be quite irritating and frightening if you worry about Alzheimer's disease. (More about that coming up.) Ordinarily though, these memory glitches are usually the result of memory inefficiencies rather than an underlying memory disorder. A memory misfire we can all relate to sometimes happens when you take a trip to the mall. After a couple of hours of shopping you head back to the parking lot—but where did you park the car? Are you parked in the row parallel to a telephone pole or was it near the third shopping cart return? Did you park in the blue section or the red section? If you draw a complete blank, one of two things has happened.

In the first place, you may not have encoded or stored the information. Perhaps your cell phone buzzed just as you pulled into your parking space and you were so engrossed in conversation on your way into the mall, the information about your car's location never made it past your sensory filters into short-term memory. If you were extremely distracted, it may not have even have made it into immediate recall. Other times, there is simply nothing particularly memorable about where you parked your car for your brain to latch on to. In either case, you didn't forget the information—because you never really learned it in the first place.

A second possibility is that you're having trouble retrieving the memory about your parking spot. The information is in your head somewhere; you just can't get to it. When this happens, you can try searching for clues by re-tracing your steps. If you were fortunate enough to encounter something out of the ordinary on your way into the mall, like some construction taking place, this will often serve as an effective memory trigger. Locate that construction area and bingo—you're all set. At other times, for reasons that are hard to explain, the car's location will suddenly just pop into your head. This may occur after a long delay despite the fact that you've racked your brain trying to re-member where you parked.

Whatever the reason you find yourself wandering the mall parking lot in search of your vehicle, as a neurologist I don't get too concerned about these minor but frustrating retrieval issues. However, when important information frequently doesn't come back or when there are more serious memory issues such as someone forgetting they even drove to the mall in the first place, a medical evaluation is recommended.

Legitimate Concerns about Memory

In most cases of dementia, it's usually the power to form new memories that goes first. This is because the brain structures involved in short-term memory processing tend to be affected early on in the course of Alzheimer's disease and other demen-tias. Long-term memories, the ones that have been embedded more diffusely in the brain's memory, often hang on the longest and are the last to go. It's not until the later stages of the dis-ease, and damage to the brain becomes more extensive, that long-term memories are affected. This is why someone with de-mentia may not be able to remember what he had for breakfast that day (short-term memory) but can recall in detail the prank he played on his teacher when he was 12 years old (long-term memory).

I have seen how this phenomenon can be confusing for some patients and their loved ones. Especially in the early stages of dementia, memory difficulties can be misinterpreted as willful inconsideration. For example, someone with memory loss may not remember to pick up a quart of milk from the store as requested, yet remembers to buy the newspaper he's bought daily for the past 10 years. It's also why a person with advancing dementia can speak fluently about the past but can have difficulty focusing on the here and now.

So when are memory glitches a cause for concern? Here are some early warning signs to watch out for:

- Repeatedly asking the same question
- Forgetting common words or mixing them up with each other
- Getting lost while walking or driving around familiar places
- Trouble following rote tasks such as making the bed or tying shoes
- Misplacing items in inappropriate places, such as putting a wallet in the freezer
- Difficulty following directions
- Undergoing sudden changes in mood or behavior for no apparent reason

Check Up on Your Memory

The thought of losing our powers of memory is terrifying. Memory is the essence of who we are, the culmination of all our experiences and everything we've learned over a lifetime. Too often I find people assume that memory problems automatically mean a diagnosis of Alzheimer's disease and they avoid seeking help out of fear. They will try to keep their struggles a secret or a well-intentioned loved one will help them compensate or cover for any deficits. Neither is a good idea. If you notice any issues with memory loss in yourself or a loved one I urge you to see a doctor for a proper diagnosis and treatment.

It's important for you to know that many factors affect our ability to remember and numerous medical conditions can impair memory. In other words, there are many treatable and reversible causes of memory loss. For example, depression, sleep disorders, thyroid dysfunction, stress, and medication side effects are common conditions that can masquerade as dementia. And as Kim Hackett shared in her story "B My Hero," vitamin B12 deficiency can do it too. We also know that underlying heart, lung, liver and kidney disease can affect memory. With appropriate diagnosis and treatment, memory can be improved and in some instances returned to normal.

This is why it's so important to see your doctor if you do have memory problems. You may well have a treatable condition. For those diagnosed with Alzheimer's or other forms of dementia, proper medical care is essential to ensure that any contributing medical issues are addressed. In addition, optimal supportive care will allow them to be as functional as possible for as long as possible.

You can also take comfort in knowing that some mild memory loss as the years pass is perfectly normal and is part of natural aging. As you get older, you may have more difficulty recalling names or words. You're likely to become prone to misplacing things or need to make more lists than you used to in order to stay organized. So long as these changes in memory are generally manageable and don't disrupt the ability to work, live independently or maintain a social life I don't usually get too worried about them.

Memory Tips You Won't Forget

Can you recall the three words from above that I ask my patients to remember? Most likely they were only fleetingly retained in your short-term memory. Because the words are commonplace and have no particular personal or emotional context for you, there is no reason for them to stick. On the other hand, if I asked you to envision the three words — ball, tree and shoe — using an effective memory technique, you would have no problem recalling them.

Envision the following scenario with as much detail and feeling as possible: Imagine you are holding an enormous rubber **ball**. It's three times your size and you have to stretch your arms out as far as they can go. The rubber feels slippery against your fingers and you must hold on tight — really visualize this and notice the rubbery scent as it presses up to your nose. All of a sudden, a gnarly **tree** with spike-like roots descends from above and punctures the ball so that it makes a loud pop. Feel the air brushing against your face as the ball deflates and you now find yourself hugging the rough surface of the tree. You then look up to see thousands upon thousands of dazzling **shoes** dangling from the branches. Watch them as they twirl by their straps and laces.

If you really visualized the above scenario in your mind's eye, there's a good chance those words are now locked in your memory. This is a common memory technique known as the link system. But what if you forget the first word? That's easy. All you need to do is link the first word to the task. In other words, imagine you're sitting in my office when I ask you to remember the three words. Picture me placing the huge rubber ball in your lap — it's so big you can't even see me and we are having this ridiculous interaction on opposite sides of this enormous ball. And of course, you now know what happens next.

Once you get the hang of the link method, you can remember countless items sequentially. If the next word was "whipped cream" you could picture those thousands of dazzling shoes flying off the tree and flinging themselves into a huge bowl of whipped cream. What makes this memory technique effective is that you are painting completely absurd pictures in your mind's eye. The more outlandish and unique you can make your mental picture, the more deeply it will be etched into your mind. This is because your brain is programmed to take notice and recollect things that are out of the ordinary.

As I previously mentioned, you tend to remember things that are personally meaningful, emotionally charged or particularly memorable. By converting ordinary objects into ridiculous, one-of-a-kind scenarios, you can make the mundane profoundly memorable. The key is to make the context absurd, exaggerate proportions, incorporate action and embellish with a variety of senses, including touch, taste, smell and sound. This may seem like a crazy way to commit information to memory, but trust me, it really works.

I first began honing these memory techniques while working at that waitress job I told you about. I visually decorated my customers in their food choices. This made my job both mentally challenging and, I must say, rather fun. Most importantly, I gained a valuable skill I've gone on to use in other areas of my life. During one particularly challenging class in medical school which entailed memorizing extensive amounts of information, I skipped the lectures altogether and spent my time creating preposterous drawings of the entire syllabus. I got the highest grade on the final exam. Again, I'm no memory wizard. I simply used a memory system that works for me.

It turns out that memory champions—those who compete in memory competitions and pull off amazing feats like memorizing the order in 20 decks of cards, thousands of digits and the names of hundreds of people in a room—frequently use a variation of this technique. There are whole books devoted to memory systems. If you're serious about learning more about how to sharpen recall, I highly recommend you read a few and try them out.

Of course there are other ways to enhance memory. Mnemonics, rhyming, loci methods, and reinforcing the information by writing it down on paper (or even in the air) all serve to strengthen retention. Repeating a piece of information to yourself such as the name of someone you just met at a party is a straightforward yet effective way to retain the information. Each time you repeat the name you are essentially resetting the clock on how long the data is held in your short-term memory. The more you repeat something the more "stable" the memory.

One of the most tried and true ways to improve your memory is to simply use it. In the story, "Capital of Delaware," Shawnelle Eliasen gives us a perfect example of this when she decides to test her memory along with her children. You probably don't challenge your memory skills on a regular basis the way you may have when you were in school and you were asked to memorize reams of information for your studies. Remember having to recite poems, memorize historical facts and commit mathematical theorems to memory? Stephen Rogers reminds us of this in his story "Partly Cloudy Pancakes." In the process, your memory skills got quite a workout. Many of us have stopped flexing our memory muscles, especially since we've ceded a good portion of our memory skills to electronic devices in this digital age. We no longer memorize phone numbers, addresses or driving directions.

The good news is that by challenging your memory, no matter what its current condition, you can make improvements. Like any other brain function, practice makes perfect. Using whatever memory method you choose, try to memorize your grocery list, an inspirational poem or the names of some people you just met. For a real memory booster, take a course that tests you on what you have learned. Exams and quizzes require you to truly stretch your memory skills.

Now that you understand why you can't find your car in the parking lot, here's what to do the next time it happens. Try roaming around aimlessly while randomly clicking your remote car lock. Eventually you'll hear a beep. It's worked like a charm for me on numerous occasions!

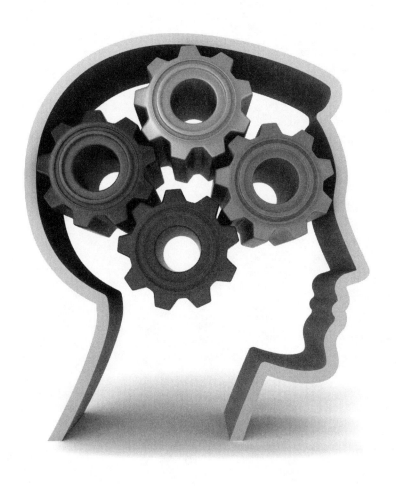

Chapter 3
Living Well to Age-Proof the Brain

Pump Up Your Brain Power

As a novelist and writing instructor, I am often asked for advice from aspiring writers. My students open their notebooks and poise their pens, hoping I'll give them some sort of magic formula to help them come up with creative ideas. Most of the advice I give, however, is pretty standard, nothing they haven't heard before: read voraciously, write every single day, study the craft of writing.

The only thing that might cause them to raise their eyebrows is my final piece of advice: exercise daily.

"You mean mental exercise?" a student once asked. "Like Sudoku?"

"I do the crossword puzzle every day," another student boasted.

"That's great, too," I said. "But no, I mean physical exercise. Something to get your blood pumping. Get your muscles moving."

My students looked at me blankly. I could tell they were thinking: We're not here to be jocks; we're here to be writers. What does exercise have to do with writing?

I understood their blank stares, because I was once in their shoes. I played sports all through my childhood and ran cross-country and track in high school, but as a busy college student regular exercise was a part of my routine that fell away. I had papers to write, books to read, club meetings and fundraisers to take part in, new friends to socialize with. Life was busier than ever. My world was expanding—I met people from not just all across the country, but from all around the world. I took an Intro to Psychology class; I learned how to play guitar; I brushed up on my rudimentary Spanish by practicing frequently with my dorm-mates. Every day, I was being introduced to literature and art and music and philosophies that I never before knew existed.

My creative life should have been flourishing, too. I should have been writing more than I ever had before. All through middle school and high school, when my days were filled with a strict regimen of class periods and after-school sports, I managed to carve out time to write: twenty minutes in the morning, half an hour before bed, one or two hours during the weekend. Ideas abounded—I was always scribbling words and phrases down on scraps of paper so I wouldn't forget any of them. By the time I graduated high school, I had published two collections of short stories, written a full-length play that was produced as my school's spring production, and was halfway through my first attempt at a novel.

In college, I was majoring in creative writing. My daily schedule, while hectic, was less structured; I may have had more homework, but I had fewer hours of class time each day. I should have been able to spend a good chunk of time dreaming up stories. I even had creative writing assignments as homework! Yet, writing was a struggle. I had dealt with writer's block before—every writer goes through dry spells at times—but this felt different. It seemed as if my creative well had run completely dry. It was difficult for me to muster the energy to sit down in front of the computer screen, place my hands on the keys, and write. My mind whirred, jumping around to class assignments I should be working on, friends I should call, what I should make for dinner, what I should wear to that party next weekend. I had never had trouble focusing before, but now I found it nearly impossible to get into the world of a story, to sink into my "writer zone."

Finally, one blustery day in early October, feeling frustrated and creatively drained, I decided I needed to get out of my cubby of a dorm room and move. So I laced up my workout shoes and went for a run. The air felt crisp and cool, and the many trees around campus were beginning to change color, their leaves blazing orange and red and burnished gold. The world condensed to the sound of my breathing, the pumping of my arms, the measured strides of my legs. For the first time since I had moved away to college, I felt calm. Like the world slowed down and I could finally hear myself think again.

Half an hour later, when I returned to my room, the blinking cursor on the computer screen no longer seemed menacing. Instead, for the first time in weeks, I felt excited to sit down and write. Ideas for characters and scraps of dialogue floated through my mind. It was like the mental pathway to my creative unconscious had been suddenly unblocked.

Now, six years later, exercise remains an integral part of my daily routine. And not just for my writing—I've found that exercise makes me feel more balanced, mentally sharp, and in touch with my emotions, which positively affects all facets of my life. Exercise keeps my creative juices flowing, helping me find solutions not just when I'm working on a story, but also when I'm faced with a teaching dilemma, struggling with a relationship problem, or feeling plagued by negativity. When I am pressed for time, I may be tempted to skip exercise for the day. Instead, that is when I know I need it most. Even a brisk walk around the neighborhood rejuvenates me and opens my mind to possibilities I had not noticed when I was hunched over my desk.

Indeed, I would argue—as Robert Frost once wrote about "The Road Less Traveled"—that exercise makes "all the difference" in the life of a successful, fulfilled, inspired writer—and person.

~ Dallas Woodburn ~

Staying Sharp at 95

I've been interested in ways to boost brain power for quite some time. I'm not getting any younger and I am finding it harder to remember names—something I did effortlessly in my youth.

The people I know who continue to have sharp minds into old age have certain characteristics in common. They are all active physically as well as mentally. Case in point, my mother-in-law. My husband and I regularly talk to and visit his mother, Lillian, a woman of 95. Up to the time she broke her hip six months ago, she was physically active. However, she has managed to adapt.

"Don't you want live-in help?" my husband asked on our last visit.

"I had help when I couldn't get around. Now I manage quite well with my walker. I need to do as many things for myself as possible," she said.

Lillian hired a cleaning lady, has food delivered much of the time, and remains living independently in the family home, a large Victorian house. Her mind is as active as ever and she is on the mend from her injury.

"Okay," she said, "let me see if I can stump you." She looked down at a sheet of paper on which she'd written questions.

Then she asked us questions she'd collected from her favorite quiz shows on television.

Over lunch, which we shared in her kitchen, I decided to interview her. "I know you never forget a phone number, anniversary or birthday. How do you manage it?"

"Simple," she responded. "I write everything down and study it. If I see it, then I can remember it." She then rattled off our phone number to prove her point.

"What keeps you young in spirit and sharp in mind and memory?" I asked her.

"For me, it's contact with family and friends. Since I can't get around the way I used to do, I talk on the telephone. It keeps me connected. I also sit out on the front porch and observe what's going on in the neighborhood. I particularly like to watch and listen to children playing. Sometimes neighbors drop by and visit."

My mother-in-law, besides being feisty and strong-willed, is very interested in people. It keeps her going. Talking to her children, grandchildren and great-grandchildren also keeps her mind active and agile, as does watching game and talk shows on TV. She feels connected to what's happening socially and politically in the world. Human interaction is a crucial element in keeping her mind sharp and boosting her memory.

She frowned at me because I was serving the lunch we brought to her house. She stated she wanted to order in from a restaurant and treat us as guests. We would not hear of it. We like to pamper her when we visit. We shop for her. My husband does minor house repairs. We bring pictures of her great-grandchildren.

"Do you do anything special to keep your memory sharp?" I asked her.

"Every night before I go to sleep I recite the alphabet backwards."

On a number of occasions, I've taken my mother-in-law to her doctor for a checkup. Lillian's doctor has observed that genetics and lifestyle both enter into whether or not a person will eventually suffer from dementia or Alzheimer's disease.

People suffering from high cholesterol, high blood pressure and diabetes are particularly vulnerable. Scientists have found associations among Alzheimer's disease and high blood pressure, which can damage blood vessels in the brain. So controlling high blood pressure is also important. My mother-in-law does, in fact, take medication to control this problem. And she watches her dietary salt intake as well. Seniors also have to be careful of drug interactions, which can affect their memory and thinking.

Lillian stimulates her mind with activities such as reading books and completing crossword puzzles. She's kept her mind active and curious in past years with such activities as reading, writing, attending lectures, and even gardening.

For those of us who are in good physical condition, walking, swimming and dancing are some of the activities that can help keep our minds sharp. My in-laws were active swimmers and square dancers for many years. They also enjoyed traveling to new places and meeting new people. All of these activities build cognitive reserve. A variety of leisure and physical activity has kept Lillian's mind sharp over the years.

I have observed that those who are active physically, mentally and socially show the least signs of cognitive decline. This was confirmed by Lillian's doctor, Barbara Paris, who encourages socialization and staying mentally active to keep your mind sharp. "If you don't use it, you lose it," Dr. Paris emphasizes, and she also says that committing to a sense of community and socialization are important. These are the very things my mother-in-law does each day.

"So why do you think you've lived such a long and relatively healthy life?" I asked Lillian.

She was thoughtful, running her fingers through her white hair. "Well, I believe in eating healthy foods, lots of fruits and vegetables, but not overeating. I try to be optimistic. I appreciate each day, and I keep myself as busy and active as possible. I try to find solutions for my problems as much as I can."

This is all true. Essentially, Lillian sees the glass as half-full. She doesn't harp on negative things. She also sees the best in other people. Her positive outlook on life, strength of character and determination to live life to its fullest and overcome all obstacles, keeps her mind sharp and sound. When there are problems, she looks for solutions. She doesn't throw pity parties. We can all learn a great deal from people like Lillian about how to boost our brain power.

— Jacqueline Seewald —

Use It
or Lose It

I love crossword puzzles. Well, wait a second... let me attach an addendum. I love crossword puzzles—even though I'm not good at them. I can honestly say that I have never finished the crossword puzzle in the Sunday *New York Times*, and that I rarely finish the crossword puzzle in *USA Today*. However, I still confidently attack them with my trusty pen—not a pencil—whenever I want to relax.

I'm afraid of Alzheimer's disease.

Well, wait a second again... let me attach another addendum. I'm afraid of Alzheimer's disease and I'm taking every precaution against it. Ranking first among my precautions, I have discovered that the strongest current evidence links brain health to heart health. Thus, my plan to combat Alzheimer's is to achieve a healthy heart. So I have adopted heart-healthy eating habits, like those contained in the Mediterranean diet. This eating plan includes relatively little red meat and emphasizes whole grains, fruits, vegetables, fish, and shellfish. Plus, it stresses the consumption of nuts, olive oil, avocados, and other foods containing healthy fats. Secondly, to help protect my brain, I do physical exercise for the heart—six days a week. Enough said.

And the topic of exercise leads me back to crossword

puzzles. I figure that the brain is just like a muscle—use it or lose it. So that's why I challenge my brain with crossword puzzles. However, I recently stumbled upon a very interesting component of that challenge.

I am right-handed, but a minor accident prevented the use of my right hand for two weeks. Thus, I continued my crossword puzzle challenges, but I did so holding the pen in my left hand. Immediately, I discovered how much more intently I had to concentrate—not only on the puzzle, but also on the simple task of writing with my off hand. I felt like I had discovered gold! So after my right hand eventually recovered, I continued to use my left. To this very day, I still do crossword puzzles with the pen in my left hand as a workout for my brain.

~ John M. Scanlan ~

Don't Forget to Dance

"I t's all in your head," my younger sister told me.

I rolled my eyes. "It's just the opposite," I insisted. "It's not in my head. Nothing is in my head anymore. Or, at least, there are major holes where there used to be memories."

I blame Facebook. In my early fifties, I added my maiden name to my Facebook profile, and boom! Two high school friends tracked me down. They were from two different high schools, two different cities and have no connection to each other. It was great renewing my friendship with each of them. The problem was, they both keep talking about major events that happened in our teens and twenties, and I have zero memory of those things. They remember in detail, but even after hearing them talk, no bells have rung in my memory. To me, they might as well be works of fiction, except that my parents verified that my friends are telling the truth.

The worst part for me is that, until this happened, I was completely unaware that I'd forgotten things. I thought I had a great memory. Well... except for the fact that it took me two years to memorize a chapter in the Bible. In my twenties I was able to memorize a chapter in a week.

"Now, my memory is like Swiss cheese," I told my friend.

"There are giant holes that I didn't even know existed." So much for the joy of renewed friendships.

A therapist friend of mine suggested that there might be a clinical problem that caused me to block out certain memories. I don't know about that. But I did accidentally discover a way to buff up my memory. At least, my short-term memory.

A couple of years ago, I was going through some enormous stress due to circumstances in my life. To distract myself, I decided to try a line dancing class that was offered at the local senior center. I'd already found that physical exercise lowered my stress level, and a line dancing class sounded like fun, so I joined. It was open to all ages, but most of the women who came, including the instructor, were many years older than I am.

"Okay," the instructor would say. "Let's do 'Come Dance with Me.'" That is no easy dance for beginners, yet these gray-haired women did it beautifully. That meant knowing the individual steps and remembering the sequence and getting their feet to follow in time to the music.

At first I fumbled around trying to get it right, while they danced with ease after just a quick lesson. Eventually I realized that there was a reason why they were so good, even though they were so much older. Dancing itself is a memory enhancer. It's youth giving. The brain is a use-it-or-lose-it organ, and these women had been building memory muscle by dancing, not to mention actual muscle. That class led me to enroll in other dance classes, for fun, for exercise, and just to socialize. And if my memory happened to improve, that was a bonus.

After enjoying the class for the last two years, I decided to memorize another chapter of the Bible. This time, even though the chapter was more complex and less familiar, it took only two months. Is dancing responsible for that? I'm not qualified to say. But out of curiosity I went online to see if there was any research that backed up my belief that there was a connection. There was. A study in the *New England Journal of Medicine* showed that recreational activities positively affected the minds of older people, and the number one activity cited was dancing. Dancing requires memorizing steps and sequences, and getting your feet and body to coordinate with what your mind is telling you. In other words, dancing integrates various brain functions at the same time, and according to the study, that rewires the brain and helps it regenerate. In some cases dancing can even reduce the risk of dementia.

For me, I started dancing for distraction, for exercise, and for fun. I had no expectation that it would make my brain younger, but even my mom says I seem to be turning back the clock. Recently I've added Zumba dancing. I'd like to tell you that I now remember the events from decades ago, but I do not. They seem to be gone forever. I can't change the past, but by dancing, I can protect the future... and have a lot of fun doing it.

— Teresa Ambord —

Living Well to Age-Proof the Brain

Introduction

I will always remember the first time I held a human brain. As a medical student I was taking a gross anatomy course and as part of the curriculum we were required to dissect a human body. The last step of the dissection was removing the subject's brain. This was a powerful moment for me. As I carefully cradled the wrinkly organ in my hands I realized that every thought this person ever had—every emotion, every experience, every dream—was coded within. It made me appreciate what a truly miraculous structure the brain is.

I know this is not an experience everyone will have in their lifetime. Nor is it an experience everyone wants to have. But there are times I wish everyone could get a glimpse of their physical brain. If they did I think they would take better care of it because the differences between a healthy brain and a not-so-healthy brain are dramatic. A vital, well cared for brain is free from blemishes, with a lovely, plump appearance and wide open arteries. In contrast, the brain of someone who has mistreated their brain with poor lifestyle choices looks shriveled with stiff, clogged arteries and large pockmarks.

Naturally we all hope to stay mentally sharp into old age and many of my patients tell me the one thing they fear the most is slipping into the depths of dementia. Yet most people seem to think you're born with an ageless brain or you're not and there is little you can do to influence how well your cerebral matter weathers the passage of time. This is not the case. We now understand that the way you care for your brain and the lifestyle choices you make directly impact its structure and consequently your personal risk of developing dementia.

The Seven Brain Aging Risk Factors

A large analysis published in the medical journal *Lancet Neurology* concluded that approximately 50 percent of all Alzheimer's disease (which is the most common type of dementia) could be attributable to what we doctors refer to as "modifiable risk factors." In other words, lifestyle habits largely under your control make a significant contribution to your susceptibility to dementia and the preservation of your mental faculties.

The study identified the following seven risk factors: diabetes, midlife hypertension, midlife obesity, smoking, depression, cognitive inactivity/low educational attainment and physical inactivity. The researchers also determined how strongly each of these risk factors was associated with Alzheimer's disease and the proportion of people worldwide and in the U.S. whose condition could be attributed to each individual factor. Of these, physical inactivity was the most significant potential contributor to Alzheimer's disease in the United States and the third largest worldwide.

As a dedicated advocate for the brain benefits of exercise, I have shared this study by the University of California, San Francisco investigators Deborah Barnes and Kristine Yaffe with my patients, and for that matter, anyone who will listen. There are multiple reasons why physical activity has such a dramatic positive effect on the brain. First of all, a sedentary lifestyle is associated with diabetes, hypertension and obesity, which in and of themselves are risk factors for dementia. Secondly, physical activity directly boosts blood flow to the brain, improves cognition and has been shown to measurably increase brain volume.

Putting aside low education and depression for the moment, impaired blood flow seems to be the common denominator among all the other brain risk factors. All of these conditions (diabetes, hypertension, smoking, obesity and physical inactivity) are associated with atherosclerosis, which results in diminished blood flow to the brain, limiting the oxygen and nutrients it needs to maintain a healthy structure and function at its best. The brain tips the scales at just three pounds, which is a mere two percent of our total body mass. Yet because it is so metabolically active it uses a whopping 20 percent of the body's blood flow.

When you connect the dots, it becomes increasingly apparent that heart and blood vessel health directly impact brain health. Research shows that cholesterol-clogged arteries, inflammation, and risk factors for heart disease and stroke contribute significantly to cognitive decline.

Restricted blood flow in the brain may also contribute to the cascade of events that leads to the abnormal accumulation of "neurofibrillary tangles" and "amyloid plaques" within the brain that are the hallmarks of Alzheimer's. Autopsies show that memory loss and poor cognitive function are more likely to have occurred when tangles and plaques are accompanied by narrowed, clogged blood vessels that supply the brain. The combination of Alzheimer's pathology and compromised cerebral blood flow is like a double whammy; neither alone may be sufficient to cause dementia, but together they seal the deal.

We also know that stroke in and of itself can cause dementia, not to mention other heartbreaking disabilities, including paralysis, weakness, trouble speaking, loss of vision, loss of sensation and other deficits, depending on which brain regions are affected. Stroke occurs when blood flow to part of the brain is interrupted and the subsequent lack of oxygen causes brain cells to die. Arteries become blocked by atherosclerosis and blood clots that arise from inflamed arterial plaques or an unhealthy heart. Keeping your cardiovascular system healthy will help protect your brain from both stroke and dementia.

While it's never too early to start thinking about brain health, it's also never too late. I think Jacqueline Seewald's 95-year-old mother-in-law Lillian, described in "Staying Sharp at 95," is a terrific role model for aging minds; when she could no longer keep her brain sharp in ways she used to do while she was younger, she adapted and found new ways to keep her brain active. So even if you have lifestyle risk factors for Alzheimer's, you can do a lot to diminish the negative brain effects. The place to start is by making an appointment with your doctor to discuss how highly motivated you are to do everything possible to decrease your chances of developing dementia.

Medical care and preventive measures for all these conditions have dramatically improved over the years and new treatments and approaches are being developed every day. I hope you will take advantage of the medical expertise that's available to ensure that you're doing everything within your power to maintain a healthy brain. Fortunately, the most effective treatments for these conditions don't come out of a lab, aren't expensive and require no prescription. Two proven ways to lower your brain risks are available for immediate use by everyone.

Nourish Your Neurons

If you need to fix a bunch of undesirable health trends like high blood pressure, high blood sugar and excess belly fat, have I got a diet for you! Following a Mediterranean-type diet can decrease your risk of Alzheimer's, prevent stroke, boost your mood, and improve cognitive function.

In 2011, Greek and Italian researchers combined the results of 50 studies that included more than half a million men and women. Overwhelmingly, the group of studies supported the idea that adopting and sticking with a Mediterranean-type diet improved blood sugar profiles, body mass index, blood pressure, and a host of other important health measures. Numerous other studies show that a Mediterranean-type diet is associated with better cognitive functioning, lower rates of dementia, improved mood and a decreased risk of stroke and cerebral vascular disease.

Note that I refer to a "Mediterranean-type diet." That's because these studies didn't look at a single, rigid diet plan outlined in some fad diet book, but rather an eating pattern that shares these general characteristics: It's low in saturated fat and high in fiber. Fruits, vegetables, whole grains and legumes are the mainstay of every meal and make up the lion's share of food items. Olive oil, which can account for up to 40 percent of daily calories, is an essential component. Small portions of cheese or yogurt are usually eaten each day. Fish, seafood and nuts are dietary staples while poultry and eggs are served less frequently. Red meat makes an occasional appearance on the menu. Small amounts of red wine are typically taken with meals though the jury's still out on whether this contributes or detracts from the overall brain benefits.

One reason this type of diet may be neuro-protective is that it's rich in mono-unsaturated fats and omega-3 fatty acids, the kind of "good fat" found in olive oil, fish, and nuts, which are the type of fats that seem to prevent the buildup of amyloid plaques in the brain and provide protection to the blood vessels that supply the brain. Conversely, low levels of dietary omega-3s and high levels of "bad" saturated and trans-fats are linked to an increased incidence of Alzheimer's.

Olive oil specifically seems to confer special benefits compared to seed oils like sunflower, soybean and rapeseed that are also high in mono-unsaturated fats. Higher consumption of olive oil has been associated with better cognitive performance and lower stroke rates. I encourage my patients to substitute olive oil whenever possible and personally use it for everything from frying eggs to dipping lobster.

A Mediterranean-type diet is also rich in omega-3 fatty acids, which is truly the closest thing there is to a miracle brain nutrient. The brain is nearly two-thirds fat, and the fats in your diet literally become the building blocks for your brain. Numerous studies have linked dietary omega-3 intake to improved blood flow, increased brain cell growth, enhanced mood, better memory and lower rates of Alzheimer's disease. Omega-3 fatty acids are found most abundantly in fatty fish, but also in fortified eggs, soybeans, and a variety of nuts and seeds. Eating fatty fish twice a week will ensure that your brain is getting an ample supply. If you can't eat fish, consider taking fish oil supplements. As always, be sure to check with your doctor first.

Eating plenty of fruits, veggies, legumes and whole grains, which are low in sugar and packed with phytonutrients is another key dietary goal. Phytonutrients is the umbrella term for all the beneficial chemical compounds found in plants, fruits, vegetables, legumes and grains that promote healthy blood vessels and reduce oxidative stress and inflammation in the brain. In addition, plant-based foods tend to be naturally high in potassium and magnesium, two nutrients that help lower blood pressure. From navy beans and red lentils to oranges and broccoli, the distinctive colors of plant-based foods are derived from their phytonutrients. Eating a wide array of colorful foods ensures that you get a variety of nature's best anti-aging and brain-boosting benefits.

My one note of caution on following a Mediterranean-style diet is to watch the sodium, which can increase blood pressure. This way of eating can include foods high in salt, such as salt-cured olives, capers, and anchovies. Instead, season foods with a variety of spices and herbs which are generously endowed with phytonutrients.

The Best Brain Booster Ever

I hope I can encourage you to take advantage of exercise, the most potent brain booster of all. It is guaranteed to enhance the very structure of your brain, improve your memory, uplift your mood, protect against stroke and decrease your risk of Alzheimer's disease.

Moving your body on a regular basis is quite simply the most transformative thing you can do for your brain. Just ask Teresa Ambord, who in "Don't Forget to Dance," found that regular dance sessions helped sharpen her memory. It's better than any pill, prescription or over-the-counter supplement for preserving and enhancing the structure and function of the brain and keeping your blood vessels healthy. It has the power to improve the cognitive function of any person of any age regardless of their past health history. In fact, its potential impact on how well the brain works appears to be greater than any other single life-style element because of its multiple beneficial effects. It directly increases brain blood flow, boosts brain volume and promotes the proliferation of new neurons. In addition, it has the power to successfully reverse and diminish stroke and Alzheimer's risk factors including obesity, diabetes and high blood pressure by decreasing long-term risk factors that thicken arterial walls and decrease blood flow to the brain.

Vigorous cardiovascular exercise gets the blood pumping to feed the brain more oxygen and nutrients. Over time, regular exercise leads to an increase in the density and size of capillaries surrounding the neurons, thereby enhancing blood flow even while at rest. One of my favorite studies to share with patients clearly demonstrates how physical activity can measurably increase brain volume. Study participants age 65 and older were asked to perform stretching exercises, continue with their routine lifestyle (which did not include significant physical activity) or walk for one hour three times per week. MRI scans of the brain were done at the beginning and at the end of the study. After six months, those participants who walked showed a visible increase in brain volume while the other two groups showed no change.

One of the potential mediators of these exercise-induced brain benefits appears to be brain-derived neurotrophic factor, otherwise known as BDNF. Released during exercise along with other brain growth factors, BDNF has been shown to boost the growth of new neurons and fortify existing neurons. It also enhances "synaptic plasticity," the ability of neurons to talk to one another, which is essential for learning and mental flexibility.

Even a single aerobic workout has been shown to increase attention, prime the brain for learning and improve mental processes. I was fortunate to realize this at a young age and used it to my advantage throughout college and medical school. My best studying was done after returning from a dance class, riding my bike or working out at the gym. I still rely on exercise to sharpen my concentration, trigger creative thinking and expand my thought processes. In fact, most of the ideas for this book were conceived and written after an invigorating run.

You may be wondering how much exercise is enough to reap all of these amazing benefits. The truth is, no one really knows. The walking study I mentioned above entailed brisk walking for one hour, three times a week. Most experts recommend getting at least 2.5 hours of weekly moderate-intensity aerobic activity, such as brisk walking, water aerobics, playing tennis or ballroom dancing. In addition, I personally recommend that you try to weave as much physical activity into your day as possible. If you're currently not exercising regularly, ease into it, but aim high. If you do exercise regularly, make it more challenging by increasing the intensity and/or duration. As always though, check with your personal physician first.

Don't let a negative mindset prevent you from working up a sweat. If you perceive exercise as drudgery and something you've failed at in the past, reframe your attitude. Reflect on the times in your life when you enjoyed moving your body. Perhaps it was dancing at a friend's wedding, playing tennis or taking a walk with a loved one? It doesn't matter how long ago it was or what you were doing. This reflection can help you understand what type of physical activity you naturally enjoy.

I do hope you can discover the pure joy of moving your

body. Every day I encounter patients who are physically handi-capped and struggle to perform physical tasks many of us take for granted. Witnessing their determination and perseverance to overcome these challenges is deeply moving. The simple act of placing one foot in front of the other is nothing less than a miracle. And for those of us who possess the ability to move, it is a priceless reminder to cherish and celebrate this gift.

If you truly want a healthy brain, exercise is simply the very best thing you can do to keep it vibrant and decrease your risk of dementia and stroke. As the Lancet Neurology study indicates, physical inactivity is the number one risk factor for Alzheimer's disease in the United States. We also know that aerobic fitness is associated with better cognitive performance and that elderly people who begin exercise programs experience significant im-provements in cognitive functioning. The fact that you are reading this book tells me you are motivated to boost your brain power. Now is the time to make a commitment to exercise. Do it for your brain.

Save a Brain

While I hope the above measures will protect you from ever having a stroke, it's nonetheless important to know the signs and symptoms of stroke. This informa-tion may help save your brain or that of a loved one. Below are a series of questions to ask if you are with someone you suspect might be having a stroke. During a stroke, brain cells are dying, so the sooner the person receives medical attention, the greater the chance of recovery. Even if stroke symptoms disappear within a few minutes, the risk of stroke is still high and you should call 911 immediately.

It's heartbreaking to see patients with neurologic disabilities that could have been prevented had they only known the symptoms of stroke. I hope you will commit to memory the five signs of stroke listed below.

Walk Is their balance off? Are they dragging one leg?

Talk Is their speech slurred? Are they using inappropriate words?

Reach Is one side weak or numb? Ask the person to raise both arms. Does one arm begin to fall down?

See Is their vision clear or partly lost? Is the person seeing double?

Feel Do they have a severe headache that peaked in severity within seconds? Do they normally have headaches? If so, is this headache different from their usual headache? Does this feel like the worst headache of their life?

*Adopted from the American Academy of Neurology guidelines

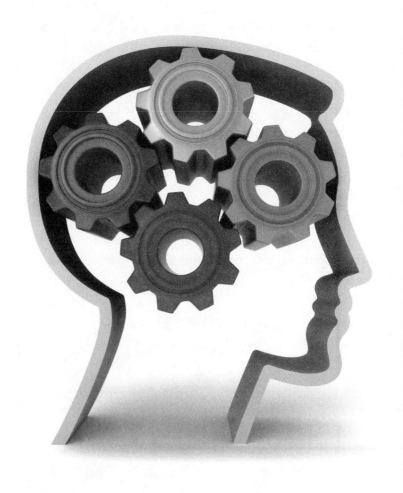

Chapter 4
Shaping Your Thoughts and Emotions

The Numbers Game

I've always loved words—their sounds, shades of meaning, and how the images they conjure can transport me to exciting places. When writing, my options are nearly limitless. I can modify verbs with adverbs, adjectives, or prepositional phrases. I can choose from a tempting array of punctuation marks as if they are chocolates on a silver tray.

Numbers, on the other hand, always cause me trouble. They slip and slide around in my brain like greased pigs on Jell-O, and I never can hold onto them long enough to do anything productive. It doesn't matter what kinds of numbers—addresses, ages, PINs, or pages. I can't even remember a new phone number long enough to dial it without peeking.

At church, when I was young, we'd be well into a hymn's second verse before I found the right page. Had the song leader said number 324, 243, or 432?

In arithmetic, numbers leave no wiggle room. Two plus two always equals four. Mathematical computations are either correct or they aren't. In desperation I've become an under-the-table finger counter. If need be, my toes can also get involved.

But I've learned to cope in daily life. When cooking, I count measurements out loud as I add ingredients. Otherwise, ringing telephones or interrupting children distract me, and I don't remember where I left off.

Instead of trying to divide odd lengths of inches by two when sewing or doing home projects, I simply pull a string across the span and fold it in half. Voilá! The exact length without frustration.

I memorize addresses by association. The first three digits in my new house number are identical to the street name where I once worked. The last two digits are the same as the final two in a familiar zip code. Such aids give me handholds until the numbers lock into my mind as a new word: fivesevenninetwoone.

I use pencil, never a pen, to maintain my checkbook register because I've been known to transpose digits, add withdrawals, and subtract deposits. I'm nothing if not creative when it comes to making errors.

In spite of coping mechanisms, sometimes I'm caught off guard, like when I applied for a new credit card and then left for a family reunion. In the middle of helping relatives fix dinner, I received a call on my cell phone from a representative wanting to verify my identity. "When were you born?" she asked.

I gave her the date.

"How old are you?"

I wanted to retort, "Honey, I gave you my birth date. You figure it out." But credit card companies have the same sense of humor as airport security guards, so I bit my tongue and tried to think. This was not a good time to be wrong.

I don't mind telling people how old I am. Every new day is a gift from God. The problem is, I have trouble remembering how many gifts God has given me. Just about the time I get a handle on the number, it changes. Fortunately, I was born smack-dab in the middle of the century, so if I can remember the current year—and my toes aren't busy—I can usually figure it out.

Most people don't understand. If I had a nickel every time someone suggested I could work with numerals if I just put my mind to it, I'd have oodles of coins. I wouldn't be sure exactly how many, but I'd be rich.

Then everything changed when I heard about dyscalculia, a learning disability with numbers. What a relief to finally have a name for my problem! I exhibit many of the symptoms: mentally mixing up numbers, having trouble remembering specific facts and formulas, and confusing similar digits (e.g., 7 and 9 or 3 and 8). Those of us with dyscalculia are often good in reading, writing, verbal skills, and creative arts, but math is traumatic for us. We can also have difficulty with rapidly changing physical directions in aerobic, dance, and exercise classes.

Studies show that dyscalculia runs in families. (It practically gallops in mine.) My mom, sister, daughter, and I have all learned how to compensate so we don't look like idiots.

But when I got a new job a few years ago, dyscalculia nearly caused me to get fired on my first day. In the interview, I answered the question about my greatest fault by saying I was a workaholic. Then I added that I had dyscalculia. The boss had never heard of it. "It's a numbers dyslexia," I explained.

She wasn't concerned. "We're strong in people with math skills. We need what you've got—writing, editing, and speaking abilities."

Relieved, I showed up the first day ready to write and edit. Instead, I was asked to count newsletters in each zip code grouping for bulk-mail purposes.

Not feeling I could refuse my first work assignment, I sat at the folding table, muttering under my breath about how I could have produced the newsletter from start to finish, but I was counting copies instead. Working my way through each stack twice, I added the results. When the sums didn't agree, I tried again, taking the two best answers out of three. Finally, I announced the total.

The office manager nearly fainted. "We're missing hundreds of newsletters!" she gasped. "Where did they go?"

I assured her there was no need to panic. Perhaps I'd miscounted. I went over the figures again. The number was higher than before, but we were still short.

By now, the office manager needed oxygen.

I could see I was likely to set a record for shortest tenure of anyone in the organization's history. But on my third attempt, I discovered that when I'd used the clever shortcut of leaving off final zeros to make columns easier to add, I'd forgotten to replace them in the total. Fortunately, the boss had a sense of humor. "Well, you did warn us." And no one in the organization ever asked me to count anything again.

The close call helped me decide to improve my grasp of numbers, so I took up Sudoku—a puzzle, based on logic instead of math, that uses the numbers one through nine. I became hooked. When I made mistakes, it was because handwritten numbers appeared totally different to me from formally printed ones. Focusing on open-topped fours written in pencil prevented me from noticing preprinted closed-top fours—and vice versa. "Maybe I can teach myself the difference," I thought.

After two years of patient puzzle-solving, I have now conquered Sudoku by treating each digit as a set of twins. That produces a total of 18 numbers to juggle at once.

Frankly, I'm amazed at my progress. But what's even more astonishing than watching slippery ciphers firm up in my brain is the confidence I've gained. I'm no longer as intimidated. I've learned that if I remain calm when standing nose-to-nose with big, hairy numbers, no one gets hurt.

I used to play games with numbers in order to cope. Now I use number games to change my brain. And who knows? Someday I may even try counting newsletters again.

~ Diana Savage ~

Slug Club

"Hey Christine, how's it going?"

I looked up from my bubble of self-pity and let my soggy pizza slip back on the cafeteria tray. I found myself eye to eye with a high school sophomore, my age, wearing a pair of crooked green glasses that magnified his eyes.

"Fine," I muttered, glancing nervously at the nearby table of "jocks" who had been my so-called friends. "What do you want?"

The boy, Brandon, who seemed to fit the labels of both "kind-of-cute" and "nerd" at the same time, thrust a flyer into my hand.

"Come join the IQ Elite at Junior Mensa Club," he said, pushing his glasses up his nose. "We meet every Tuesday, and we will prevent you from becoming just another teenaged mental slug. Did you know a baby octopus is about the size of a flea at birth?"

"Interesting," I said, with as much enthusiasm as possible, hoping he would go away. "I'll think about it."

As he left I felt another wave of self-pity envelop me. Ever since my knee had been injured in a basketball game my sports had gone out the window—running, swimming, biking, basketball... everything. I was an outcast from my friends. An enraged outcast. And if even the nerds were taking sympathy on me, I was obviously falling pretty low on the social ladder.

I looked at the flyer.

"Come join Junior Mensa! To participate you must pass a basic IQ test, memorize 50 interesting facts, dedicate yourself to a minimum 15 minutes of classical music studies a day, and be taking a language course. We meet every Tuesday, but keep exercising your brain all week!"

I crumpled the flyer into a ball and put my head on the table. Sure, I might be a mental slug. I subscribed to the theory that intelligence was unhealthy in excess quantities. The most brain power I used was calculating my mile splits when running around the track.

Yet as we were dismissed from the cafeteria and I saw my friends receding in a tight group, I found myself unconsciously smoothing the flyer out again. In the rage I felt for being abandoned I suddenly saw Mensa as a challenge—just like any challenge in sports. Who was to say I couldn't pass a stupid IQ test and memorize 50 facts? Who was to say I couldn't learn a foreign language if I wanted to? Who was to say I couldn't—at least until my knee got better—become a temporary "nerd"?

That evening I Googled everything I could think of related to improving mental prowess. I even made a list of my brain's workout regime. Every afternoon I assigned myself the task of completing two puzzles and two crosswords in less than one hour. Afterward I was to listen to 30 minutes of Mozart while memorizing trivia from the Internet. Then I had to study all my textbooks.

Meanwhile, I was also going to have a strict lifestyle change. I had to limit my junk food intake (it restricts brain cells from growing), skip items with simple sugar (insulin is released into the blood and makes a person sluggish), get a minimum of eight hours of sleep, and drink one cup of coffee every morning (the caffeine is an ideal mental stimulant). It was going to be tough, but I felt up to the challenge. After all, it couldn't be any harder than running mile repeats in Track. I vowed to knock the socks right off the Junior Mensa team.

At first the regime seemed impossible, especially when I saw my old friends trooping towards the gym for basketball practice after school. Yet this only made my competitive fire burn brighter. At lunch I started eating a deli sandwich with skim milk, and for desert I had a tub of vanilla yogurt. I realized I felt more energized, and for once, intelligent. Did you know that Teflon is the slipperiest substance in the world? Or that medical research has found substances in mistletoe that can slow down tumor growth? Or that lemon drops are as acidic to your teeth as battery acid? I was brimming with knowledge.

When the time came for the Junior Mensa test I approached Brandon with as much self-confidence as humanly possible.

"I'm here to take the Junior Mensa test," I said self-importantly. "Do you want me to recite my 50 random facts or take the IQ test first?"

Brandon was surprised.

"Oh, you wanted to do Junior Mensa?"

"Yeah...."

"We didn't have enough people interested, so we had to cancel," he said.

I felt as if I was an insignificant ant that had been stepped on. My mouth dropped open as I realized that I had just wasted three weeks of my life becoming smart... for nothing.

I went home that afternoon in a daze, and found myself unsure of what to do with myself. Eventually, following my old routine, I set to work solving crosswords and creating puzzles. What was I doing this for? Fortunately, as the last note of Mozart's "Symphony 25" hung in the air, I had an epiphany.

"Slugs..." I said thoughtfully. "Teenaged mental slugs..."

The next day I made a beeline for Brandon at lunch.

"I think I know what's wrong with Junior Mensa," I said, ignoring the stares from his "nerd friends." "It didn't have enough relevance to real life... How many times in your lifetime do you need to know that a hippo can open its mouth four feet wide?"

He didn't answer.

"Exactly. Trivia means nothing. Learning should be about making decisions that improve your life... keeping your brain active reduces your risk of dementia; reading improves your memory and vocabulary; doing sports decreases stress and risk of depression with endorphins. It's relevant to everyone, not just nerds. Here." I handed him a flyer. On it I'd written, "STOP THE SLUGS!"

After a second, a grin spread across his face. He agreed to meet me at school the next morning and start distributing posters. Among the "STOP THE SLUGS" posters were signs on healthy eating, proper sanitation, exercise, and, my personal favorite... a poster of gorillas that said "Cliques are primitive. Start the evolution!"

To begin recruiting members we handed out free coffee

that had been donated by the teachers' lounge, with signs that illustrated the mental benefits of caffeine and its stimulation. We also recited the benefits of getting at least eight hours of sleep. In our first week we recruited 150 members—nerds and non-nerds. Brandon and I, who were now widely recognized as the ringleaders, suddenly found ourselves being treated like school celebrities. But most important to me was the day when my old friends, the "Jocks," walked over to greet me.

"Hey Christine, that SLUG stuff looks like it's gotten really big," my old friend Callie said.

I nodded. "It has. We're trying to make brain improvement a goal for everyone, regardless of social status."

"Urm... well... do you think we could join?"

I grinned in disbelief.

I knew at that moment that I had finally reached my goal. To this day, though I am now capable of doing sports again, I no longer consider myself a primitive member of the "Jocks," nor a trivia-memorizing member of the "Nerds." Those fences have been shattered. My pride for what I have done—improving the minds of teens, breaking social barriers, and creating awareness of lifelong learning—is greater than the pride I felt winning any sport. The Slug Club, our high school society that encourages lifelong learning and good decisions, lives on.

~ Christine Catlin, age 17 ~

The Handkerchief Caper

I've spent my adult life as a college professor teaching people how to think more creatively and use more of their brainpower. My college writing textbook is based on over 100 brainteasers that help people maximize their abilities. Interestingly, this lifetime passion was awakened by a casual contest when I was a child.

At a family picnic for employees of the company where my father worked, they held contests for the children—who could blow the biggest bubble-gum bubble, who could hop the longest on one leg, who could throw a softball the farthest. I was 13, full of enthusiasm and the spirit of competition, so I threw myself into the contests. The grand finale, the handkerchief-throwing contest, I realize now, was not meant to demonstrate any real skill, but simply for laughs. But it stirred my love of thinking outside the box.

The emcee gave each of the dozen children a cloth handkerchief and told us the winner would be the one who threw it the farthest. The first throwers, the little ones, took mighty wind-ups, but when the cloth left their hands, it opened and fluttered to the ground a few inches in front of them. The next kids threw harder and harder, but with no better results. The crowd roared with laughter, and being 13, I didn't like adults laughing at us. The older the children, the more the crowd laughed at the feeble results.

It was obvious that using the same technique would not work. I didn't understand anything about wind resistance or density then, but I did know that a rock would fly a lot farther—far enough to break a garage window, I knew from bitter experience. Suppose I tied a rock inside the handkerchief? No, it was "throw a handkerchief," not a rock and a handkerchief. When they inspected it, I'd be disqualified. If I knew anything about adults, it was that they lived by rules. There were rules for eating, dressing, working, watching television, even rules for sleeping. And they loved to pounce on a child who violated them. I was the one who climbed fences and who tried to dig to China. "You'll break a leg" and "It can't be done" just rolled off my back.

So it irritated me to see the kids throwing harder when the handkerchief always opened, caught the air and died. The secret was not to throw harder but to keep the cloth from opening. Suppose I hid a rock in the cloth without tying it. The rock would drive the cloth at least farther than the others, and when they separated, people might not notice a small rock landing in the grass. I had a good chance of getting away with it, but I didn't want to win by cheating. What I really wanted to do was show them that a kid could beat them at their own game. I had to make the handkerchief fly like a rock. Like a rock! That was it! I began tying the handkerchief around itself to make it small and compact, like a rock. I secretly tied knot after knot until it was the size of a large walnut. When I approached the line as the final contestant, there were a dozen squares of cloth littering the ground. People were already chuckling, anticipating a big strapping boy like me hurling it a few inches.

I took a long wind-up, and the balled handkerchief rocketed off into the trees maybe 60 feet away. The laughing died in a collective gasp. The emcee stared at me with narrowed eyes and then ran to retrieve my missile to expose how I'd doctored it.

He came back slowly. "It's just the handkerchief," he declared, holding it up and untying the knots. The adults applauded good-naturedly, and I felt cocky. But it was more than that. Adults believe they can control kids—and each other—through rules. But all rules have loopholes and I'd just discovered that real thinking means finding them.

"That's not fair," a man said. "It's cheating."

"He threw the handkerchief," the judge said with a shrug and a grudging smile. "We didn't say he couldn't tie it."

I had not broken the rules, but I had broken the preconceptions of the rules, and that, I learned from this contest, was the secret to creative thinking. If you want to maximize your brainpower, you can't accept rules at face value. Oh sure, people who want things to turn out predictably will be upset when someone sees different possibilities. The man who grumbled could not let it go. "I still say it's cheating," he hissed at me. "You think you're so smart."

Well, I was 13, so he was probably right about that. I pasted an innocent expression on my face, even though I was dying to tell him my back-up plans: I could have thrown the open handkerchief and then flapped my baseball hat or puffed at it to make it go farther. I could have rolled the cloth around itself instead of tying. I could have soaked it in cola for extra weight. If I'd had time to starch the cloth, I would've folded it into an airplane like you do with paper and sailed it.

This moment started my career of thinking. I was thrilled with my little victory over regimented thinking. I wanted to continue looking beyond what things seemed to be. To live creatively, you have to tap into the less-used parts of your brain, and not accept stereotypes, slogans and unquestioned ideas. I wish our business and political leaders would try this. I wish people in stale relationships would try to break the artificial rules that strangle them. If things are not going well, you can't keep responding the same way.

— Garrett Bauman —

Don't Overload Your Brain

D o you want to maximize your brainpower? Spin every plate that comes your way and juggle all the jobs you can handle. That would have been my advice just a short time ago. I was a multi-tasking mama! My perspective changed after I was rear-ended on the interstate. As a result I suffered a traumatic brain injury that changed my life forever. During the first days and weeks following the accident, I used words inappropriately, my emotions were out of control and my memory came and went. The brain that I had relied on as a source of independence and strength was failing me.

I was prescribed months of cognitive therapy and rehabilitation that would eventually help me function at normal levels again. I was encouraged to use online math games and many organizational tools and I was taught to use constant reminders, lest I forget or lose anything because of my memory problems.

I found many of the resources provided to me to be invaluable, but from all of the lessons, one seemed to stand out to me above all the others. I learned that it was important for me to slow down and take my time while my brain was healing—it was therapeutic for me.

As I reflected on this, I thought of how my teenage children get frustrated with our computer when it is running slowly. Instead of patiently waiting for it to load, they repeatedly click the mouse and other buttons until the computer locks up completely and has to be shut down and restarted.

I realized that I often treated my brain the same way. I would load it with multiple projects, deadlines, committees and activities. When it didn't perform, I didn't slow down my pace; instead I was likely to add in some form of self-improvement plan in an attempt to fix my brain. More times than not, I would encounter a season of burnout or sickness that would set me back much longer than if I'd simply slowed my pace. When I chose not to take care of my brain, it eventually caught up with me and required a shut down and restart, much like my overloaded computer.

I've since recovered from my brain injury and am back to work, but it's a constant temptation for me to take on too many tasks. Despite those temptations, lightening my load has not only been good for my brain, it's been a gift to me. Today, I am able to relax. I can simply watch a television program without working or reading during the commercials. I've learned that living in the moment is all about retraining my brain to focus on one thing at a time. Now when my kids have something to say to me when I'm on the computer, I take a break from my typing and look at them until they're finished speaking. Previously, I would've convinced myself that I was having a valid conversation with my kids. I say "no" to many more things than I used to, but I say "yes" to my family, evening walks, special projects that I'm most passionate about. I experience much more peace these days and I know my brain thanks me for it.

~ Stephanie Davenport ~

Shaping Your Thoughts and Emotions

Introduction

I think most people have the impression that thoughts and emotions pass through their brains like the weather, sometimes floating about on a gentle breeze while at other times raging through the mind on the gale force winds of a hurricane. And, like the weather, it may seem like the only thing you can do is passively listen to the day's forecast and hope for the best. Actually, there's a lot you can do to influence how you think, which consequently will determine the way you feel.

The Physical Path of Thought

Ideas and feelings exist in the brain as a series of electrical and chemical reactions. Brain cells, known as neurons, "talk" to one another by sending messages back and forth through the spaces between them called synapses. A thought travels through the brain when signal-sending neurons release neurotransmitter chemicals into synapses and receiving neurons pick them up. It is estimated that the human brain contains 100 billion neurons, each of which has thousands of connections to other neurons.

On average, each connection transmits about one signal per second, with some specialized connections sending up to 1,000 signals per second. All in all, the remarkable communication network in your brain is a maze of trillions upon trillions of connections capable of performing 20 million-billion transactions per second.

This is a somewhat simplistic explanation of a very complex process we don't completely understand—and may never fully understand. However, thanks to brain imaging technology, scientists have a pretty good idea which areas of the brain are associated with which types of thinking and they can reliably track a lot of thoughts and emotions as they speed through the intricate neural networks.

We now understand that thoughts are structurally encoded within the brain. Every time you think a specific thought, specific pathways of neurons fire up. With repetition, these pathways are strengthened. The more often you think a specific thought, the more well defined the path between neural Point A and neural Point B becomes. Over time, you develop habitual thoughts and predictable reactions because it's convenient for the brain to send ideas down well paved, clearly marked highways rather than little used side streets. The brain, being a creature of habit, when left to its own devices, quite literally prefers the path of least resistance.

What Is Your Inner Voice Telling You?

The chemistry and electricity of thought I just described

translates into an ongoing internal dialog that streams through your head from the moment you wake up in the morning until the moment you lay your head on the pillow at night. Everyone has one, this inner voice. It provides a running commentary about how you think and feel about both yourself and the world at large. Listen carefully and you'll find that this voice has a habit of repeating the same automatic thoughts over and over. In the process, these pathways are becoming stronger and more ingrained over time.

Unfortunately, the things your inner voice says to you aren't always kind or in your best interest. Yours, for instance, may spend a lot of time chattering about mistakes or inadequacies that make you feel bad or dwell on people and situations in a negative way. It may discourage you from trying new things by telling you you're not good enough or continually reminding you to feel angry, sad or anxious.

The brains of people with gloomier inner dialogs seem to have a different structure and function than those with sunnier inner dialogs. Glass half full thinkers have more activity in the left prefrontal lobes of their brains, while glass half empty thinkers have more active right prefrontal lobes.

But here's the good news: Because your inner dialog is so much more than intellectual clouds and psychological mist, you have the power to change it. With focus, practice and time you can learn to redirect thoughts by reinforcing new, more desirable neural pathways. When you begin thinking new, different thoughts it literally changes the physical structure of your brain. You build and reinforce new connections within the brain and after a while your thoughts automatically tend to flow in the direction of your deliberate choosing. When this happens you will have changed the configuration of your brain and your chosen way of thinking will become your natural response.

I think Diane Savage's story "The Numbers Game" showcases this phenomenon perfectly. She could have chosen to pigeonhole herself as someone who was bad with numbers but instead she decided to think of herself as someone who could improve a weakness. Even though she struggled with dyscalculia, a learning disability related to numbers, she didn't let it define her and she didn't let it stop her from finding novel ways around it. That's positive thinking.

Minding Your Brain

Our growing understanding that modulating the tone of internal dialog actually does rewire the structure of the brain comes from groundbreaking research. Studies done at Massachusetts General Hospital and Harvard Medical School document actual physical changes in the brains of people who made a conscious effort to adjust their automatic thought patterns through meditation.

The researchers reported on a group of subjects who, as part of a stress reduction workshop, were asked to meditate an average of 27 minutes daily. The volunteers practiced a form of meditation known as mindful meditation, which involves observing the thoughts that run through the brain without judgment. The goal of this practice is to become more in touch with what's happening in your mind and body in the here and now and carefully listening to your inner voice. When you experience a distressing thought or emotion you learn to identify its true nature and give yourself the choice to think and feel differently.

One of the most advantageous things about mindfulness is that it allows you to step back from your inner dialog's self-criticism and recognize it for what it is: self-sabotage. Instead of repeatedly reinforcing unproductive thinking, you learn to stop negative thoughts in their tracks and forge new self-enhancing neural pathways.

After eight weeks, brain scans identified noticeably increased thickness in structures associated with focus, attention, memory and learning and some of the areas associated with compassion, introspection and self-awareness. No brain differences were observed in the non-meditating control group, which led researchers to believe the changes they saw couldn't be explained away by the simple passage of time.

On a behavioral level, meditation appears to improve the powers of attention and focus. This in turn helps regulate impulsiveness and creates a greater awareness of repetitive, self-defeating thoughts. Once you recognize a propensity for negative thinking, you can work at replacing it with a more affirmative, uplifting thought process.

Of course, mindfulness meditation is just one technique that can teach you to avoid fruitless mind traps. It can be very effective but it's not for everyone. I know plenty of people who've never set foot in a yoga class or meditated, but who have successfully improved the tenor of their inner voice. Perhaps prayer, physical activity, gardening or playing the piano is more your cup of tea. I encourage you to discover what works best for you and begin to take charge of your brain.

You Are What You Think

So why should you make an effort to send your thoughts in a more upbeat or calmer direction? It turns out that the general trend of your habitual thinking affects your life on many different levels. Did you know, for example, that optimistic people are actually luckier? Thinking good thoughts won't increase your chances of winning the lottery—too bad!—but an optimistic frame of mind does seem to be better at spotting possibilities and opportunities.

In one study, participants were asked to count the number of photographs in a sample newspaper. Subjects who described themselves as "lucky" were much more likely to notice a message on page two, disguised as a half-page advertisement with large block letters: STOP COUNTING—THERE ARE 43 PHOTOGRAPHS IN THIS NEWSPAPER. The researchers surmised that the "luckier" individuals paid more attention to their surroundings, which made them more apt to notice the message in the newspaper. They were also more likely to be extroverted, open-minded and optimistic, personality traits that appear to up a person's "luck" quotient.

Neuroscience is now beginning to understand that your inner voice has a profound effect on your overall physical well-being too. It influences your day-to-day health, how susceptible you are to illness and disease, and even how long you live. In fact, cutting edge work being done by Harvard and Massachusetts General Hospital demonstrates how the way you think affects you all the way down to the cellular level.

The research team trained subjects to perform the "relaxation response," a technique developed by Dr. Herbert Benson, a pioneer in mind/body medicine. The relaxation response is a state of deep rest that changes the physical and emotional response to stress. Their goal was to see if this training could alter a person's gene activity and change the "expression" of genes related to stress and inflammation. After just eight weeks of relaxation instruction, the subject's gene expression profiles changed dramatically. Among the subjects in the relaxation response group, roughly 2,000 genes active in various stress-related physiological pathways had been deactivated. In other words, Dr. Benson's group has shown that we can literally reprogram our cells by altering the way we think. To me, this is one of the most important studies in the field of neuroscience as it provides scientific proof of the mind/body connection and the profound realization that we can choose to improve our health by redirecting our thoughts.

Chronic stress takes a toll on the brain. Cortisol, otherwise known as the stress hormone, has been shown to be toxic to neurons in the hippocampus, the brain's memory center. Animals under chronic stress have smaller hippocampi and studies suggest that the same holds true for humans. According to one study, people prone to distress were nearly two and a half times more likely to develop Alzheimer's disease than those who weren't. We also know that those who suffer from anxiety and depression have an increased risk of Alzheimer's and stroke. Learning to de-stress and improve your frame of mind not only makes you feel better, it has the power to improve your brain and your overall health.

Optimize Your Inner Voice

I hope you will take the time to begin paying attention to your own inner voice. If you have positive thoughts, hold on to them like treasures. However, if your inner voice tends towards the negative, be reassured that you have the power to retrain it. Everyone has the ability to change their brain and in turn change their attitude—and vice versa. If you feel you'd benefit from a bit of neural fine tuning, know that you can make real, measurable adaptations to your brain and that it's never too late to start. In my profession—and in my own life—I've seen people make dramatic improvements using a variety of methods to take control of their thoughts, behaviors and emotions. It all comes down to discovering what works best for you personally.

Meditation, relaxation training, biofeedback, yoga and cognitive behavioral therapy are some of the approaches you can use to tune into your inner voice and begin modifying it to serve you better. You can do it on your own, but if you don't feel you're making progress, I would encourage you to seek out a professional instructor or licensed therapist. Often, the hardest part is getting started, because we're so used to listening to that inner voice which says, "you can't change me." But any little bit of time you can carve out for yourself, where you stop juggling a thousand things and stay still for a moment of self-reflection will begin to reshape your brain towards more positive thinking. The simple act of listening to what your inner voice is telling you can be invaluable. At the very least, it's important to tune into the conversation in your head so you know what your brain is up to.

Don't stop there. There's no reason to accept the heavy price you pay for succumbing to a self-defeating mindset. Practicing relaxation techniques and taking charge of your thoughts will allow you to gain control over your mind and consequently, your life. You can then apply these skills to overcome issues like weight problems, depression, phobias—whatever you want to improve in your life. In the process, you'll discover the true power of your mind.

5-Minute Mini-Meditation

Try this mini meditation session to give yourself a few moments of quiet reflection each day. I think you'll find it's worth the investment.

Sit in a quiet, comfortable place, where you won't be distracted, with your back straight and your hands resting in a comfortable position. If you wish you may conjure a higher power to help give meaning to the experience. Gaze gently downward so that you aren't focused on anything in particular. If your eyes become heavy, let them close. Allow your breathing to become deep and rhythmic. If your attention drifts a bit, so be it. Don't worry about whether you are "meditating the right way." Your aim should be to simply clear your head and relax. Even if it's just for a few minutes, that's okay. The most important thing is to get started and go easy on yourself. With practice, your ability will improve. The payoff is so tremendous, it is well worth the effort.

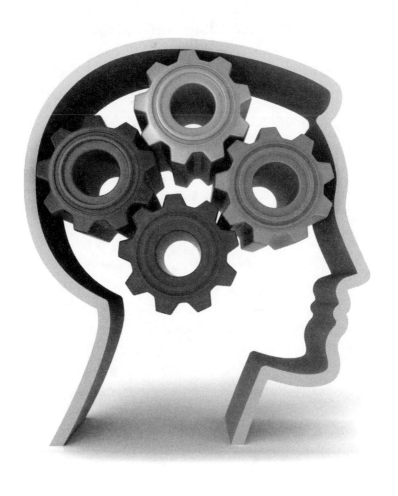

Chapter 5
Wake Up
Your Brain

Nothing Beats a Good Book!

I t was *"Pop" Warner's Book for Boys*. I'll never forget it. I was probably around seven years old when my parents gave me that book. Who could have guessed what a fire it would light in my life?

Thanks to old "Pop," I was encouraged to develop a passion for sports, a habit of clean, upright living, and most of all—to fall in love with books. When he told me, in his book, that athletes never drink, smoke, or swear, I believed him! And I made sure I never did, either. Books can have a tremendous influence, especially when it comes to raising the bar on our thinking and behavior.

I'm known as a voracious reader and usually have several books going at one time, with a goal to finish one every day. Each one has made me a different man than I was before I opened it, but a few have made a profound difference in my life. I think particularly of *Veeck as in Wreck* by the late great Chicago White Sox owner Bill Veeck—a book I discovered while working in the Philadelphia Phillies organization. Thanks to a fortunate set of circumstances in my life at that time, I had the opportunity to meet Veeck. We developed a lifelong friendship, and few people have had a greater influence on my NBA executive career.

By the early 1980s, I found myself receiving numerous requests to speak before audiences at a variety of venues. I was flummoxed. What kind of message could I deliver? How could I develop the confidence to speak with conviction? Could I, little ol' Pat Williams, actually make a difference in others' lives? I knew I'd find the answers I sought in books, and I was not disappointed. Two wonderful volumes, both written by longtime NFL defensive end and ministry founder Bill Glass: *Expect to Win* and *Plan to Win*, laid out the principles I needed to launch my speaking career.

Today, I speak on a regular basis. And everywhere I go, I issue my reading challenge: one hour a day, from a book. I don't care how you do the hour—it can be 60 minutes all at once, two 30-minute sessions, four 15s, or 60 ones. Just do it! When you make that commitment, you'll be finishing an average of one book a week. That's 52 books a year! The very idea sends an endorphin rush straight through me.

In the research done for my book *Read for Your Life: 11 Ways to Transform Your Life with Books*, we came across data corroborating the brain-boosting power of books. One report suggested that such mind-engaging activities as crossword puzzles and reading can actually delay or even prevent age-related memory loss. Another article from a renowned health professional touted the importance of keeping our minds from wandering. I don't know about you, but I plan to live every day with a sound, fully engaged mind, and nothing I've found keeps me more focused than a good book.

As a reward for my reading evangelism, I regularly receive

letters, phone calls, and e-mails from those who've taken up my one-hour-a-day challenge. They feature key words and phrases like: "Your book has transformed my life!" "I am honored to accept your challenge to read every day" and "books have allowed me to educate myself... to become more confident, to become a better conversationalist, and have provided me with opportunity and inspiration for many of my personal projects." If that isn't evidence that reading boosts your brain, I don't know what is.

I've heard it said that reading is mental dental floss. And I believe that once you've made books an integral part of your life, as I have mine, you'll agree that nothing comes close in the brain-boosting category.

Most people who know me will say that I am something of an over-the-top kind of guy. And with my 50-year career in professional sports, my 19 children, and more than 70 published books of my own, they would be right. I believe in squeezing every minute out of every day that I possibly can. Even now that I am battling multiple myeloma, I'm doing my level best not to yield any ground. And why not?

After all, we are not here on our own time. We owe it to the one who gave us our life in the first place to put it to good use.

In my home I have a vast library of books. And at the heart of them all is that Pop Warner book—red, cloth-bound, and well worn from all the reading. Nothing has influenced me more than the love of reading that book inspired. Why not power up your brain with a great book, starting today?

— Pat Williams —

Get Out
of That Rut!

Have you ever broken your dominant arm and tried brushing your teeth with the other hand? A real pain, right?

But that broken bone was a good thing, too. Because while your arm was mending, your brain was getting stronger too. It got stronger as you learned to write with your other hand. And eat. And brush your teeth. Whenever we use our brain to make our body do things it's not used to doing, the brain gets stronger.

The giant spider web of neurons and synapses that fills the amazing three-pound organ inside our skulls gets denser and more complex. And that's a good thing.

The happy news is that you don't have to break a bone to put your brain to work learning new tasks. It's simply a matter of getting out of your rut and doing everyday things just a little differently. Here are 10 things to try, in addition to brushing your teeth with the "wrong" hand:

- Tie your shoelaces a different way.
- Watch a television show that's broadcast in a foreign language.
- Drive to work using a different route.

- Reverse the order in which you read the newspaper.
- Get dressed in the dark (but check your appearance in the light before you go out!).
- Shop at a new grocery store.
- Thread your belt through the loops in the opposite direction.
- Put your earrings on in reverse order.
- Kick a soccer ball with your non-dominant foot.
- Walk backwards for 100 steps.

After a while, doing things the new way won't seem so new—or so awkward—at all. Meaning that your wonderful brain has trained your wonderful body to unfamiliar tasks. Now it's time to give it more challenges. Like learning to play a musical instrument. Or counting to 20 in Mandarin Chinese. Working the New York Times crossword puzzle. Writing poetry.

Your brain muscles will thank you for the exercise. As they grow stronger every day.

~ Jennie Ivey ~

Book Brain

After I gave birth, it seemed my brain had been yanked out of my body along with my newborn son. In those next weeks, everything became a murky fog, with calendar dates blurring and conversation threads lost in mid-sentence. The mental lapses made sense while I coped with middle-of-the-night feedings. "Oh, it's just 'mommy brain,'" other women would say with a laugh, relating how they left the store with groceries on their car roof, or showed up for an appointment on the wrong day with the wrong kid.

However, months passed. Little Nicholas began to sleep through the night, yet I remained in a constant state of confusion. It didn't help that my sailor husband was often stuck on ship for long stretches at a time, leaving me to manage the house on my own. The days were a blur of diaper changes and feedings, with the occasional outing for groceries or a game night at a friend's house. And the game nights weren't that much fun when I could barely add 2+2 without pausing to think about it.

I told myself that I'd start to feel competent and intelligent again after Nicholas was a year old. Then I said I'd have time for myself after my husband returned from deployment. Then he returned, but was still kept busy on the ship for days and weeks at a stretch. I was still muddling along in my mommy brain-fog. Enough was enough. No more excuses.

I thought about my life pre-baby, pre-marriage, and then, pre-college. What brought me joy? What made me engage my brain?

I wandered through the house and found hundreds of answers staring me in the face: books.

Back when I was a kid and a teenager, I used to go through a book a day. Contrast that to the past year. I had read about five books, and bits and pieces of others. A lot of those books had been about pregnancy and babies, not the escapist historical fiction and fantasies I used to love. The problem was, I didn't sit down and read like I used to. I didn't know how to find time during the day, as everything revolved around Nicholas. By my bedtime, I was so tired that all I could do was sit in front of the television and vegetate.

I looked online, and on LiveJournal I found the exact motivation I needed: the 50 Book Challenge. Read at least 50 books in a year, whatever subject or genre I wanted. Members could post book reviews on the community, creating a huge database of new and old books to recommend or revile.

This was what I needed, a brain-booster that didn't involve price comparisons on diapers. Goals always worked well for me—give me a deadline, and I can get a task done. For a long time I hadn't had any ambition other than to sleep, eat, and keep the kid clean and happy. Now I had a goal of my own.

I began to follow the online community and within days I discovered new books of interest. I compiled a wish list, and ordered some fresh reads. I tore apart my bookshelves and organized the books I already owned so I could start whittling my way through my unread stockpile.

January 1st arrived. I had my resolution for the year: 50 books, and no excuses. I started reading.

A few days into the year, I saw someone had already read five books. Wait, what? I was already behind? No way. My competitive spirit kicked in.

I found time where it had never existed before. I read as my son watched *Sesame Street*. I read as I ate lunch. If I rode the bus, I brought a book in my purse. I read as I stirred pasta for supper. I read before bedtime, even if it was just a few pages. I brought my own books to doctors' waiting rooms so I wouldn't squander time on magazines.

My brain awoke from hibernation. I could recall what I did on a certain day or week, simply by remembering the book I read at the time. And I admit, for a long stretch I was the dreaded stay-at-home mom who could only talk about her kid. Now I had new and exciting things to discuss, whether it was the latest bestseller I learned about in a review, or my newly completed read about the settling of the western United States. At my moms' group, I struck up a friendship with a fellow reader. We talked books and new releases and favorite authors.

Then my son Nicholas started joining in.

He knew his letters and numbers, and he began to recognize the black squiggly lines in the books I read aloud to him. He saw his mommy reading—and obviously enjoying what she was doing—and he began to bring me armfuls of books.

"Read?" he'd ask in his hopeful little voice. Therefore, it only made sense that when he was two, the very first word he read on his own was "BOOK" on a store sign.

I had started out with a selfish goal to bring my own brain back to life. I did that, and more. I showed Nicholas the joy of reading. Reading also became a habit and wasn't something I squeezed into the day. If I sat in a chair for more than a minute, that meant I needed a book. Nicholas began to do the same.

Now it's not uncommon for my lanky first-grader to bring a stack of books to the couch and stretch out for an hour or two of reading. I sit in a chair nearby with a cat in my lap and a book in my hand.

We're together and reading, and all is right with the world.

~ Beth Cato ~

Practice
Makes Perfect

I didn't think much about it at first. I would be listening to someone and find that my mind would wander a bit from time to time. Suddenly, I would realize that there was an awkward silence. The other person was waiting for a response and I had no idea what they had said. It was very embarrassing.

After apologizing several times for "zoning out" during a conversation, I realized that I needed to do something about this problem of mine. It was like I had developed attention deficit disorder. One day I accidently stumbled down the right road to a solution.

I was sitting in a doctor's office, flipping through the reading material, when I came across one of those word search books. It was the kind where there is a grid of letters on each page with words hidden within the grid. You had to find the words by searching the grid. I was completely engrossed in one of these puzzles when I was called back to see the doctor. Wow! I had focused on something so completely that my name had to be called more than once.

After the visit, I went to a local bookstore and picked up several of these word search puzzle books. There were many variations on locating the words in the puzzle, but I found I enjoyed them all. In the beginning, I just started with the first word in the list, then searched the grid until I found it. This was very time consuming.

Having worked through an entire book, I began to develop tricks to find the words. I would group words that began with the same letter and search for them all at once. This speeded up my search since it reduced my passes through the grid. Then I realized that some letters were easier for me to spot than others. For instance, I can spot O, U, M, W, C, I, and L easily. So I began to group words that contained these letters.

Of course, there were several different types of puzzles. I could not use my new tricks to solve them all, but I developed other techniques for these. The important thing was that I was giving each puzzle my full attention. I was focused. I never left a puzzle undone. I always completed it before I put down my pencil. I never looked up answers in the back of the book. I stuck with it until I solved it.

One day I picked up a book to work a puzzle and something interesting occurred. I found that I could just look at the puzzle and the words would almost leap off the page at me. I found them quickly, zipping right through the puzzle. It startled me a little. I tried another one with the same result. I realized that I had trained my mind to recognize the patterns that made up common words. I began to notice that I was more focused on conversations. There were no more of those awkward silences. I felt happier and more confident.

I also realized that in the old days I had sometimes read the same line in a book several times before I focused enough to actually retain what I had just read. That seldom happened anymore. It was true. You can teach an old dog new tricks!

I thought back to younger days when I would sit and practice the piano for hours at a time. Then one day, I realized I could play the songs without the sheet music in front of me. I had not deliberately memorized the piece. My hands had been trained, from repetition, to move over the right sequence of keys.

I began to remember how constant practice in sports had improved my game. I had trophies for shooting from the free throw line in basketball because I practiced the shot hundreds of times. I could hit the basket in my sleep. I could put a ball in exactly the same place over a tennis net for the same reason. Repetition.

Somehow, I had lost sight of that simple lesson that so many teachers and coaches had instilled in me for years. Practice makes perfect. I don't do word searches as much as I used to. I have moved on to simple video games. When I master one, seeing the pattern or the path to winning repetitively, I move on to something else.

I plan to keep building those neural pathways in this old brain of mine, always searching for new challenges. Hopefully, it will serve me well for many years to come.

— Debbie Acklin —

Lullaby and Good Night

I was 42 years old and I wanted to cry like a baby. I was so exhausted that I couldn't even stay awake sitting in a restaurant with friends. I couldn't drive for fear of falling asleep behind the wheel. The last time I had been out in public, I had taken my grandmother to her cardiologist and had fallen asleep in the waiting room, only to wake myself with my own outrageously loud snoring. I was mortified! "Grandmother, I snored in front of everyone!" I shouted—in front of everyone. They all laughed, as did my granny, and I survived the humiliation because of the graciousness of these strangers, but I knew something was terribly wrong with me. I struggled so hard to stay awake just doing ordinary things—talking to my students, singing in the church choir—that I was miserable.

I went to bed at night like everyone else, but after the lights went out, all bets were off. I woke gasping for breath more and more often. I was filled with terror. "I'm going to die!" I told my doctor. I started sleeping sitting up on the edge of the bed. It was excruciatingly uncomfortable. Every time I nodded off a bit I jerked upright to save myself from falling. But to relent and lie down was to risk that horrible inability to breathe.

Everything bad in life is made worse by the simple lack of sleep. A writer and a tutor, I found I couldn't concentrate.

My memory failed. I forgot simple things, like how to define "gerund," and whether or not I'd fed my dogs that morning. My brain was dying from the utter lack of sleep.

I finally relented and went to a pulmonologist who specialized in sleep disorders. He had an immediate handle on the issue.

"Sleep apnea?" I asked when he offered the possibility. "What's that?"

People with sleep apnea stop breathing in their sleep. When they stop breathing, their brains react and send out alarms. The body hears those alarms and jerks awake. People with sleep apnea suffer from fragmented sleep because their brains are not allowed to relax into a deep restorative sleep. This can cause heart and lung problems if left untreated.

If sleep apnea was my real problem, and my doctor was sure it was, I could only ignore it at my own peril. Despite my misgivings and fear of hospitals, I relented and had a sleep study.

Anyone who has trouble sleeping in his or her own bed knows full well that sleeping with electrodes glued all over one's head, eyes, chest and legs in a strange bed is not the recipe for sweet dreams. To make matters worse, nine o'clock was the "suggested" lights-out time and I almost never went to bed before three or four in the morning.

The findings were conclusive: I did, indeed, have sleep apnea. In fact, I stopped breathing as many as six times a minute. I was horrified to get this news. I might have cried at learning my diagnosis had it not been tempered with some very good news: sleep apnea is absolutely treatable. I had seen the ugly, sci-fi-looking CPAP machines in my pulmonologist's office. This machine would push room air into my airway as I slept, forcing my windpipe open, keeping me breathing, and allowing me to stay asleep rather than be constantly jerked awake by a brain alarmed that I was going to suffocate. I was a bit daunted by the ugly facemask, but I was not dissuaded. Other people might choose nighttime beauty over rest, but not me. I was excited about the chance to sleep soundly while the machine kept my oxygen levels high. I would finally be able to wake each morning with a clear head. I was fitted for a full facemask and went voluntarily back for a second night of sleep study so my machine could be calibrated.

The following day I said a tiny "hallelujah!" as the medical supply woman arrived at my house to set up my CPAP. "Now, try the machine for at least a month before you decide it won't work for you," she warned. "It's a hard thing to get used to."

But it wasn't. I knew before the woman even left that getting used to the machine was not going to be an issue for me. I was so, so tired. I was polite and I walked the woman out, but I nearly bounded back into my bedroom after I closed the door behind her. I sat down on my bed and placed the mask on my face as I'd been taught. The machine, sensing my breath, turned on automatically. I knew the air pressure would keep me breathing. For the first time in over a year, I slept for two solid hours. It was the best sleep I'd ever had.

That evening, I wrote a story and sold it the next week

without even a second draft. I immediately felt like myself again. My memory functioned normally. I could read books!

Looking back, I'm surprised at how long it took me to seek medical help for my sleep problems. Getting my CPAP was the best thing that had happened to me in a long time, and using it made my entire life feel "right" again. I still use it nightly. My dreams are sweet.

~ Marla H. Thurman ~

Wake Up Your Brain

Introduction

In medical school I used to do my best studying right before lights out. If I had a biochemistry test I would hit the books right up until bedtime, then drift off to sleep where the vivid molecular structures I had just studied would creep into my dreams. I would wake up with those molecules committed to memory, ready to ace my exams.

This experience was one of my first inklings of the amazing powers of sleep. Now as a practicing neurologist, I have worked with patients and reviewed studies that confirm my belief that the sleep and rest we often take for granted are so very important for the health and functioning of the brain.

Sleep to Remember

In retrospect, my vivid molecular dreams make a lot of sense. Research indicates that sleep does indeed reinforce learning and is crucial for consolidating memories. Studies also show that dreaming about a problem will help you solve it. To get a picture of what goes on in our heads as we slumber, researchers place a series of electrodes on the scalp to record the electrical activity of the brain. This machine, known as an EEG, gives scientists a window into the distinctive rhythms of the sleeping brain and has helped us understand the cyclic stages of sleep.

Every night your brain goes through four to six sleep cycles. Each cycle lasts about 90 minutes and is composed of four stages: a dream stage called REM (rapid eye movement) and three stages without dreaming called non-REM. The deepest stage of sleep occurs during non-REM and is called "slow wave sleep." This appropriately named stage is characterized by a dramatic slowing of brain wave frequency. Many of the restorative benefits of sleep appear to occur during this phase.

In contrast, during REM or dream sleep there is heightened brain activity. In fact, brain metabolism is greater during REM than when we are awake and actively concentrating on a problem. During REM we appear to run through the events of the day, which is thought to aid in solidifying new memories and learned skills. Dreaming also seems to play a role in fostering creativity and inspiring new ideas. It's important to know that just because you don't remember your dreams, it doesn't mean you're not dreaming. During REM sleep, it appears our memory centers are busy processing information from our awake hours rather than actively recording what is happening in our dreams. Therefore, you will only recall a dream if you wake up during the dreaming phase of sleep.

While we don't fully understand the purpose of dreaming or slow wave sleep, we do know that adequate amounts of both are critical for learning and optimal brain functioning. For example, studies by Matthew Walker and Robert Stickgold found that after a good night's sleep, a newly learned motor skill will show a dramatic improvement in accuracy and execution without any additional practice. While the biggest jump in sleep enhanced learning occurred after the first night of training, further improvement was noted after two consecutive nights of sufficient sleep. Study participants who were deprived of a full night's sleep after training and those who were taught a skill in the morning and then retested 12 hours later showed no improvement in their performance. This is one of my favorite studies to share with patients who skimp on sleep, especially students who think pulling an all-nighter before an exam is a good idea. And whenever a patient complains of memory problems, I always consider inadequate sleep as a potential cause.

What You Lose When You Don't Snooze

Beyond improved memory, concentration, reasoning and mood, scientists agree that sweet dreams are critical for maintaining a healthy brain and body. Recent studies suggest that sleep enhances the proliferation of new neurons (neurogenesis) in the hippocampi, (the brain's memory centers) while sleep deprivation reduces the production of new neurons in these regions. Additionally, it appears that beta amyloid, a byproduct created by cellular activity, which accumulates in Alzheimer's disease, is cleared from the brain during sleep. This may explain why other studies show a link between sleep deprivation and Alzheimer's disease. Sleep also provides the brain with a chance to stock up on energy sources, neurotransmitters, growth factors and cell-building proteins it has gradually used up during waking hours.

Besides taking a toll on the brain, lack of sleep or poor

quality sleep has widespread detrimental health effects, including impaired immune function, weight gain and decreased pain tolerance, along with an increased risk of high blood pressure, diabetes and heart disease. We also know that sleep deprivation disrupts the normal secretion of hormones that regulate and maintain bodily functions. For example, human growth hormone, which repairs and rebuilds tissues throughout the body, is primarily secreted during deep slow wave sleep. So if you're not getting enough sleep, you're missing out on the closest thing there is to the fountain of youth.

Brain scan studies also show that chronically short or interrupted sleep brings on profound changes in the emotional centers of the brain. These areas shift into overdrive as they cease to communicate coherently with the parts of the brain involved in logic and reasoning, which are themselves also functionally compromised. This may explain why overtired people tend to fly off the handle with little provocation. In severe cases someone who is habitually unrested may develop depression or anxiety. It is almost as though, without sleep, the brain is unable to put emotional experiences into context to produce controlled, appropriate responses.

Even in the short term, the brain doesn't appreciate being deprived of rest. Though some people report feeling a buzz or even a sense of euphoria after pulling an all-nighter, they may not realize just how loopy their judgment and decision-making abilities become or how severely basic cognitive functions like planning, focus and attention are impaired. One night's sleep debt can reduce daytime alertness by more than 30 percent.

A perfect example of this can be found in driving statistics that attribute one out of five motor vehicle accidents to drowsy driving. Australian researchers found that being awake for 18 hours straight produced impairment equal to someone who is legally drunk. And just like someone under the influence of alcohol, sleepy drivers are not aware of the risk they take when they get behind the wheel. Missing one or two hours of shuteye on a given night makes you twice as likely to be involved in an accident as someone who has had a full night's rest. Lose more than three hours of sleep, and the risk of falling asleep behind the wheel increases five-fold.

For all these reasons it's easy to see why sleep is so essential, especially for keeping the brain humming along. It's clear that neglecting sleep isn't a great idea. Taking steps to correct poor sleep habits and to address underlying issues that lead to insomnia can do amazing things for your brain and overall health.

Slumber Numbers

There doesn't seem to be a way to train the brain to go for more than a day or so without sleep or ask it to function properly on less sleep than it needs. That said, a good 40 winks does seem to restore the balance of communication between the brain's reasoning and emotional areas after a period of sleeplessness. (As we discussed above, it's a different story for memory.)

So how much sleep is enough? I wish I could give you an exact amount but I can't. Most experts agree that the average person does best with between seven and nine hours a night but there doesn't seem to be one magic number that's right for everyone.

Sleep requirements, like food preferences and personal style, are highly individual. That said, most Americans aren't getting enough sleep, but they don't realize it because being sleep deprived has become their normal way of life. Over the past 50 years, the average night's sleep for adults has dropped dramatically, from more than eight hours to just over six and a half. Perhaps the best indicator as to whether or not you personally reach your ideal sleep number is whether or not you feel rested and refreshed when your alarm clock goes off and have the stamina to make it through the day without taking frequent coffee runs or nodding off at your desk.

Part of the problem with arriving at an optimal sleep number is that it's not just about quantity. Sleep quality is also important. We've all experienced restless nights where we log enough sack time, but nonetheless feel lethargic in the morning. On these nights your normally rhythmic sleep cycles become fragmented and your brain is deprived of the restorative slow wave sleep or REM sleep that is necessary to feel refreshed.

Many environmental factors disrupt sleep. Culprits range from a partner's snoring to a lumpy mattress. More commonly though, personal health issues such as frequent urination, bodily pain or discomfort, acid reflux/heartburn, and hot flashes in women are to blame. A wide variety of medications — as well as alcohol, caffeine and nicotine — can alter the natural rhythm of your sleep cycles, leaving you groggy in the morning.

Sleep disorders such as "restless leg syndrome," which causes an irresistible urge to move at night and obstructive sleep apnea (OSA) are common causes of daytime drowsiness. In OSA, just as the body fully relaxes and the brain slips into deep sleep, oxygen levels plummet due to airway obstruction. Low oxygen levels trigger alarms for the brain to wake up and breathe, yanking it from the brink of sound sleep. Often those with OSA are not even aware that they suffer from the condition as they may not fully awaken. More commonly, a bed partner will notice loud snoring and sudden, brief pauses in breathing during the night. Over time, untreated OSA can cause serious lung, heart and brain dysfunction. Fortunately, Marla Thurman knew this. In her story "Lullaby and Good Night," she recounts how getting treatment for this condition improved her life immensely. So if you think you or a loved one may have OSA, it's very important to see your doctor.

Finally, as we all know, anxiety and stress are two of the most frequent causes of tossing and turning at night. It's common to have occasional bouts of insomnia due to short-term stress, family concerns or looming deadlines. However, when sleeplessness occurs for months on end, it's considered chronic and a medical evaluation is warranted. The reason you can't sleep could be behavioral, environmental, emotional or medical. Or it might be a combination of issues. If you can't resolve your sleep issues with any of my suggestions from this chapter, make an appointment with your personal physician and consider seeing a sleep specialist. You deserve to enjoy all the important benefits good sleep has to offer.

Tips for Better Sleep

- Keep to a regular bed and wakeup schedule even on the weekends.

- Create a comfortable, dark, quiet environment that is conducive to sleep. (If necessary wear earplugs and/or a mask.)

- Don't eat a big meal before bedtime or go to bed hungry. If you must, eat a light snack that's high in complex carbohydrates to promote drowsiness. Avoid alcohol, caffeine, and nicotine close to bedtime.

- Address recurring sleep disruptions including your partner's poor sleep habits and/or snoring. Getting help will mean a better night's sleep for both of you.

- Expose yourself to bright light first thing in the morning to regulate sleep/wake cycles. If you live in a place that's often overcast, consider purchasing a light box.

- Dim the lights in the evening and avoid bright, fluorescent lights to enhance the release of the sleep hormone, melatonin. Replace bright light bulbs with low-wattage bulbs in lights you use frequently in the evening.

- Avoid watching TV or using computers and other electronic devices close to bedtime. The blue light they emit suppresses melatonin release.

- Address medical issues that disrupt sleep such as frequent urination, pain, acid reflux, hot flashes, restless leg syndrome and obstructive sleep apnea (OSA).

- Exercise regularly—it is one of the best ways to ensure you sleep deeper and longer. If possible, engage in outdoor physical activities to boost the sleep benefits even more.

- Many common medications can cause insomnia and disrupt normal sleep cycles, including antidepressants, blood pressure meds, asthma meds, decongestants, steroids and stimulants. Review your medication list with your doctor to see if there are alternative medications or if it's possible to rearrange your medication schedule for better sleep.

- Similarly, many medications can cause drowsiness and

so are best taken at bedtime. As always, review with
your personal physician before making any changes.

- Consider relaxation techniques and/or cognitive
  behavioral therapy to help you fall asleep and stay
  asleep. This type of therapy has been shown to be
  just as effective as sleeping pills, but without the side
  effects. You may want to try working with a licensed
  therapist to master the skills that will be yours to
  use for a lifetime.

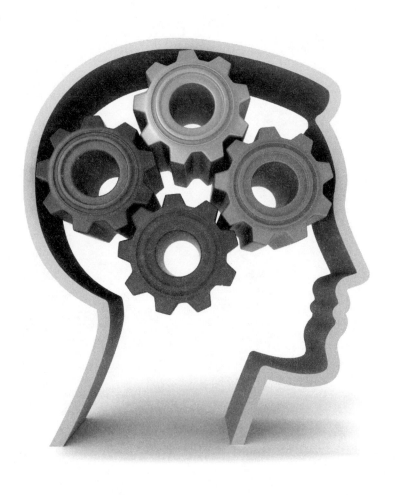

Chapter 6
Don't Accept Labels

Rise and Shine

Five months after our wedding, my wife is killed and I join millions of other brain injured Americans when a van broadsides our car at 75 miles an hour and smashes us into a tree. There's a brain injury in America every 21 seconds, a stroke every 45, making them the leading cause of acquired disability. Of the survivors, some 40 percent will have at least one unmet need a year later, so strokes and traumatic brain injuries are threats to the brain that we often don't overcome—and mine are massive.

That night, my family grieves for my wife and me, and learns how much about the brain remains unknown. Doctors tell my parents that my arrival at the ICU in the lowest level of coma they measure—a Glasgow Coma Scale 3—means that I will likely either never wake up, or die.

When, after over a month my eyes open, and my parents ask the care team what the future holds for my shattered mind, body and soul, the doctors say I might or might not get better: how much no one knows.

The medical system discharges me from outpatient therapy when I score a Full Scale IQ of 89—the lowest end of average. Once you touch average the medical insurance system moves you out, often sooner once your benefits are exhausted.

In addition to touching average, I'm also discharged because Full Scale IQ is supposed to stabilize or solidify at age eight. As I'm an adult, significant improvement beyond this point is not expected.

With a Full Scale IQ of 89, my mind works so slowly that given two-and-a-half hours to take a test that a normal person would finish in 50 minutes, on a good day I might score an "F" and fail it.

I'm designated a non-reader, with all the limitations to my mind and future that my inability to focus my eyes, read or write entail, and discharged home to my family.

Blessed with a mixture of determination and luck, they find treatments not widely known or made available, answers that yield miracles of recovery for my mind and spirit. They include craniomandibular alignment using integrated bio-mechanics and computer-enhanced graphics to affect posture, balance and muscle strength throughout my body; three-dimensional nuclear and radiological imaging of my neurovascular anatomy, and training of the processes that constitute cognitive functioning—how my brain acquires, retains and retrieves new information.

As my brain functioning improves, I realize the global scale of the threats to our mental health. It occurs to me that there should be an easier path for victims than my family's struggle to find answers, and that finding how to overcome these threats, make the most of our minds, and boost our consciousness is the greatest challenge of our times.

It slowly dawns on me that sharing my experience of recovery might help others and make a lasting memory of my wife, and this leads to the most satisfying work of my life. I write the book that I wish someone had given me at the start of my journey of recovery, filled with information and inspiration.

Its dedication reads, "For everyone who needs to find the hidden path," and *Rise and Shine: The Extraordinary Story of One Man's Journey from Near Death to Full Recovery* is compared by some to a detective thriller, as it describes how my family search for clues and answers—and insurance coverage—to restore my mind.

Rise and Shine receives perhaps a unique distinction for a book written by a patient—a full medical peer review by the highly respected *Journal of the National Medical Association*. Both reviewers praise its information as "specific" and "valuable," but raise a critical medical question—whether my brain improvement is unique to my case, or reproducible in other patients.

My opportunity to answer it comes on an international stage when an admirer of *Rise and Shine*—Lakshmi Pratury, Content Curator for the INK Conference in association with TED—flies me from Los Angeles to speak at their inaugural Conference in Lavasa Hill City near Mumbai, India.

For my INK talk on TED entitled, "Don't take consciousness for granted," I show the audience first a graph of "Patient A." This shows how, from "Untestable" during my coma, my brain processing reaches a Full Scale IQ of 89 at the time of my discharge and thereafter, with cognitive and other therapies, remarkably climbs to 150+.

Then to answer the fair question of the JNMA reviewers and show how my results are not unique, I present to the international audience results from Patients "B" and "C." They illustrate how Full Scale IQ may measurably and repeatably be assessed and optimized for youths and adults.

Now available in multiple languages and seen around the world, my INK talk on TED leads to an invitation from Deepak Chopra to present my ideas at his foundation's Sages and Scientists Symposium in La Costa, California, and interviews on National Public Radio. TED Conference organizes an online "TED Conversation with Simon Lewis" entitled, "How do we make the most of our Consciousness?"

Scheduled for two hours and extended to two days due to exceptional audience interest, it draws some 2,000 visitors, and over a hundred who participate with comments, from countries including the U.S., India, South Korea and China.

From the tragedy of my crash, my life's work changes from Hollywood filmmaker to an advocate, spreading awareness of how we may protect and raise the level of our cognition.

For my ongoing work through *Rise and Shine*, I wish to conduct a long-term population study to explore how many in society may benefit from the treatments that I describe, that changed my mind and changed my life. It will seek to depart from the normal focus on effectiveness of one specific treatment. For I believe that the outcome that matters to each of us most is the combined effect achieved by an integrated approach to the most important element within us—our overall mental processing, and our consciousness.

Do we allow some children to limp in their learning and become kindergarten (then high school, then college) dropouts, or do we use an integrated program to screen for and detect learning difficulties, prevent academic failure, and seek to optimize the mind?

The exploration I describe in my memoir, in my INK talk on TED, on National Public Radio and in online media about me is a journey that grew my mind to an extent the doctors never thought possible. It took me along "the hidden path" in ways that I hope inspire others with ideas how to transition from potential mind toward actual mind. To maximize our consciousness each day that we feel the sun rise and shine. Which is why I call my first book and exploration of how my family enabled me to rebuild my consciousness *Rise and Shine*.

~ Simon Lewis ~

My Traveling Brain

"This looks like a college dorm room." That's what my doctor said when she came to visit me in the nursing home. She was intrigued by my toys, computer, Keurig coffee maker, stacks of books, *The New York Times*, *New Yorker* magazines and portable DVD player (God knows I had to keep up with *Mad Men*!). At this stage of my life, I knew it was essential to stay connected to what was happening in the world. Most importantly, I needed to stay connected to my dear friends.

At 87, people always want to know how I stay mentally sharp. My answer is simple—friends, reading and staying mentally active. When I was young I served as a WAC during WWII. I met many people from all over the country who shared their life with mine. Living together in very tight quarters we all realized that we are one and the same. We learned so much from each other. Or at least I did. From there, I took my books and traveled into a marriage and raised two daughters.

Later on, I was lucky to work for an airline. My favorite subject in school was geography and I wish I could thank Mr. Durant, my seventh-grade geography teacher who inspired me to travel. I have seen much of the world on the cheap. Believe me when I tell you, we airline people know every inexpensive pensione on the face of the earth (and heaven too!). Although I never went to college, I've always loved to read and I've always been curious to learn new things. My books, adventures and the people I have met throughout my life have given me the best education I could ask for.

Everyone thought I would stay in the nursing home for the rest of my days. With the help of my daughter, my friends and lots of determination, I eventually moved into my own apartment. They tell me I'm the only nursing home resident they know of who was under hospice care and actually left on my own two feet. I found some secondhand furniture and once again moved all my toys. I even got a cat from a local shelter named Sheba. I can look out my balcony and see the ocean. With my books, computer and DVD player, I am as happy as a clam at high tide.

The only traveling I do these days is on my computer. If I hear about a new place, I'll look it up and learn everything I could ever want to know about it. I keep in touch with the friends I have made over my lifetime by phone, e-mail and on-line. (Though I must say, I've yet to friend another octogenarian on Facebook!) I've made new friends at my apartment complex—one of whom helped me type this. I have had ups and downs, health issues, sad times, but more funny times. Unless it is a real tragedy, most situations have a belly laugh, which makes everything better. I also have a new collection of pals. I joined the knitters and craft group in my medical day care program, which I attend one day weekly. There are six women who are very busy crocheting hats, blankets and tiny little slippers for the newborns in a Boston hospital. In 10 months I have three inches of a scarf to show for my efforts. But it is the conversation and companionship that I enjoy. Life is certainly different, but I am comfortable, happy and still curious. Who could ask for more?

— Anna (Betty) Brack —

Just a
Little Farther
to Go

Nothing she was about to say could possibly shock me. I figured the test results would confirm what we already knew, but that didn't make hearing the news any easier.

Sure enough, reviewing the file, Gina said, "John's memory skills are at the level of a child four years and eight months old. In other areas, John's brain is functioning like that of a seven- or eight-year-old."

I glanced over at John. At 6'5", my son was hardly a child. He was, in fact, 34 years old and the father of two precious boys. As the vice president of our family-owned chain of convenience stores, he'd been a real go-getter, taking us from 17 to 36 stores. My husband called him a genius.

Then one Sunday our lives changed forever.

While riding his motorcycle without a helmet, John was blindsided by a car. Flying 150 feet, he broke his pelvis in three places and suffered massive head injuries. He spent the next 70 days in a coma, plus nine months semi-comatose where he couldn't talk and could barely respond.

Home now for six months, John couldn't remember

anything longer than a minute. He got disoriented if left alone even briefly. He couldn't taste or smell, his peripheral vision was gone, and he saw everything through what he described as a watery tunnel. And conversations were close to impossible. He had no "filter," interrupting constantly and talking loudly non-stop, expressing every random thought lest he forget it.

We had driven five hours to meet with Gina, the director of the San Antonio center of LearningRx, a brain training company that helps people with TBI, strokes, autism, ADHD, and more.

I let what she'd said soak in. Then I asked. "Can this help John?"

She said, "Scientists have learned that the brain can physically reorganize itself—even rewire neural connections and create new ones—our whole lives. That's what we're counting on for John."

We knew about brain training. John had signed up with a company offering online brain games, which had improved how he tracked things with his eyes. But we needed so much more.

Gina was offering us something completely different: personalized one-on-one brain training, plus professional testing to measure improvements. A trainer would take John through targeted mental exercises to strengthen and re-grow connections in his brain.

"A computer program can be turned off," Gina explained. "But we're going to push John, just like a physical therapist would push him physically. Plus, we can do things that a computer program can't."

Initially, John needed an hour of brain training daily for 12 weeks. Because we lived so far away, Gina would teach us how to do some of the training at home. Could this be the answer we'd prayed for?

On the long drive back home to McAllen, Texas, I reflected on all that had happened over the past 18 months.

It all began when I answered a call from my daughter-in-law and heard the chilling words, "John's been in an accident."

My husband James and I met April at the hospital. We were praying when the ambulance pulled up. As they wheeled John in, I asked a paramedic, "What can we do?"

"Just keep doing what you're doing," he said gently. "Your son's going to need a lot of prayer."

John didn't exactly "wake up" after his 70 days in a coma. Instead, he was what the doctors called "minimally conscious." He couldn't respond. He was in diapers and on a feeding tube.

By then he had been transferred to TIRR Memorial Hermann (The Institute for Rehabilitation and Research), where the staff began the slow process of trying to wake his brain.

The first thing they did was tape his eyes open, to stimulate his brain. Other days they put ice on his face or coffee grounds in his mouth, trying in vain to get a response. Then one day they pulled the hair on his forearm and he flinched. We were thrilled! It seemed cruel, but they were trying to get him out of the darkness, out of the place where he was.

One day my husband opened John's curled hand and held it. James said quietly, "I know you're in there, son. I love you so much. If you can squeeze my hand a little and let me know we're communicating, it would be cool. Here, I'm squeezing your hand three times, that means I love you. Can you squeeze my hand back?"

He told me later, "Jan, I don't know if an angel pushed that finger, but John squeezed back."

On the 335th day after the accident, John simply shot out of where he was. I was beside him when a new speech therapist walked in and said, "Hey John, who's this with you?"

He said, "Mom." We were still screaming with joy when he said, "Mom, lemme use your cell phone, I gotta call April and Dad and let them know I'm talking." His voice was raspy and rough.

Nine days later, he came home. TIRR—and God!—had accomplished a miracle! But as James says, what do you do after the miracle? What do you do after you bring someone home? How do you get them to the point where they can function, have a job, do their thing? John needed to go further.

Could brain training get us there?

John's trainers—Catherine in San Antonio and Patty at home—were determined to find out.

In an early session, John became argumentative, saying he didn't need to improve his memory.

Catherine said, "What if you need to remember something?"

"I put it in my cell phone."

"Where is your cell phone right now?"

He got quiet. Then he said, "I can't remember."

Within weeks, John started noticing when he was talking too loud and would quiet himself. As his memory improved, so did his "filter." He stopped interrupting and talking non-stop. Suddenly he could hang onto thoughts, sort them, and express what was appropriate.

One day Catherine asked him where his cell phone was. He laughed and said, "It's lying face down in the cup holder in the front seat of the car."

Before brain training, he couldn't handle even one of his children (who are three and five) by himself. If they stepped out of John's circle of vision, he couldn't find them! Now he regularly takes them fishing, or to the beach, or simply plays and wrestles with them at home.

McAllen Medical Center and Methodist Hospital in Houston saved his life. TIRR woke up his brain. LearningRx is turning him from a child back into a man. When they test his brain now, he's functioning at the level of a young adult.

John is a living miracle. Recently he told us, "My brain was like this," and he held his hands together, his fingers mashed and jumbled. "Now it's like this," and he aligned his fingers, leaving them slightly crossed. "I've got just a little farther to go."

~ Jan Keller ~

The Power of Perseverance

I had come to visit my parents on their 50th wedding anniversary. My mother was facing Dad's bed in the intensive care unit of the hospital with her back to the door. Dad lay unconscious, fast in the grip of congestive heart failure and pneumonia in both lungs. Not exactly a party atmosphere. Mom was in the middle of giving Dad a pep talk. I stood at the door and listened.

"Come on Bob, the kids are counting on us. They've planned a big party. You're a Marine. My Marine. Marines never give up. You've got to rally!"

Mom's words flowed strong and steady. Each phrase driven by her determination and punctuated by her fist raised high in the air. Mom knew just how to talk to a Marine, having been one herself during World War II.

"Fight, Bob. Fight!"

The only other sound I heard was the steady whoosh-whoosh emanating from the ventilator that was keeping Dad alive.

Mom patted his hand, then pulled the wooden rosary beads from her pocket, resolute in the power of prayer. If her pep talk couldn't rally him back then the good Lord would. She never doubted that Dad would recover.

Though it seemed impossible to me that dark January day,

Dad pulled through. But it was a full month before he made it out of the intensive care unit, and another month before he felt the sun on his face outside the hospital. Of course we put all plans for their 50th anniversary celebration on hold, though I recall my brother and sisters and I throwing a pretty good hoot and holler party in my parents' driveway the day Dad finally came home.

In the hospital we all noticed some definite issues with Dad's short-term memory, but the doctor explained that his brain had suffered oxygen deprivation and assured us that it was most likely temporary. We had no idea until Dad was home a day or two that his short-term memory loss was just the tip of the iceberg. Before long, Mom discovered he wasn't reading the newspaper. When she asked him why he said he just wasn't interested, but she suspected it was something more.

In the past, it was a rare day that my dad didn't figure out the daily cryptogram in record speed. Now he didn't even want to look at it. He had trouble telling time, couldn't write a check, and the saddest day of all was when he carried his shoebox stash of cash over to me and asked me to count it for him.

All year long Dad squirreled away cash in a shoebox and when the real estate tax invoice arrived, the shoebox of cash was emptied to put a dent in the bill. For whatever reason that always gave Dad a feeling of accomplishment.

I sat down at the dining room table as he opened the box and pushed it toward me.

"It's a lot. Isn't it?"

"Yes, Dad. You did great this year."

Tears welled in my eyes as my dad, the machinist who

thought nothing of measuring in micrometers, looked at me with the innocence of a child who could not tell a five-dollar bill from a fifty. I sorted the money and counted his bankroll. The total came to $300.

"Do you want to count it too, Dad?"

He tried. In fact he tried three times but continued to get confused and finally gave up.

"It's okay. I trust you," he said with a wink, then cast his eyes down and blushed from embarrassment.

That evening I called my mom and asked if she noticed Dad struggling with counting his money.

"That's it!" she said. "I didn't pray him all the way through double pneumonia and congestive heart failure so we could sit by and watch his brain turn to mush. The Marines have landed, Annie, and we're going to win this one."

"Right. So what's the plan, Mom?"

"Starting tomorrow morning we're not avoiding the newspaper anymore. We're going to sit down on the couch and read it together. Out loud. He can like it or not. He's going to do it. In the meantime you're going to the store and buy children's crossword puzzle books."

"I'm on it, Mom!"

I don't think Dad knew what hit him. If he asked what time it was, my mother would point to the clock and say, "You tell me. The big hand is on the six and the little hand is on the five." If he didn't get it right she'd explain the face of the clock in 15-minute increments and she'd ask again. He'd try again. It wasn't ever easy but Mom never caved.

While all of that was going on my sister Marie put together a cryptogram puzzle book for Dad that was filled with cryptograms my brother and sisters and I wrote. Each one related to our family, friends, events from the past, household calamities, favorite jokes, his favorite sports teams—anything we could think of that would jog his memory and make the puzzle solving fun.

Dad worked those puzzles and cryptograms with dogged determination. Each one he solved increased his confidence. Every morning Dad read the newspaper to Mom and no matter how many words he stumbled over, he kept at it.

For Dad the road back was quite a struggle, but by June, when he was finally well enough for us to have their 50th anniversary celebration, he was fully recovered in mind and spirit. His body was another story, but he accepted his limitations with grace and good humor.

Sitting on my night table is a framed photo of Mom and Dad. Of all the terrific candid shots my husband Joe has snapped over the last 30 years, this one is Nobel Prize quality to me. In it Mom and Dad are standing arm in arm wearing bright bejeweled golden crowns and jubilant smiles. Behind them hangs a banner displaying the phrase "Happy 50th Anniversary" in gold foil letters.

We partied in a big way that day. Mom and Dad celebrated 50 years of marriage, five children, nine grandchildren and one great-grandchild. But when I raised my glass in honor of the happy couple, in my heart it was the grit of two old Marines and the power of perseverance I toasted.

～ Annmarie B. Tait ～

Ageless
Occupation

It came as a shock when the new president of the company where I had worked for 29 years called me to his office one Tuesday morning along with the director of human resources. He opened his portfolio and announced cheerfully, "We're planning a retirement luncheon for you this Friday and thought we'd get a list of the executives you'd like invited."

As editor of the company's travel magazine I had founded some 20 years earlier, I had received nothing but glowing reports on every review.

But the truth is, I was 78 years old and highly paid. I suspect the company felt that it was time to bring in a younger person at a lower salary in this period of economic stress.

"Are there no other jobs in the company where I might fit in?" I asked, reeling in shock.

The HR director stepped in. "None at your salary," she assured me.

"I heard they were looking for a writer in travel promotions," I ventured.

"You wouldn't be interested in that. The pay is in the thirties."

"I'll take it," I said boldly. "I don't really care about the money. I just enjoy working."

The new president looked startled. He exchanged questioning glances with the HR director, then folded up his notebook and stood up.

"Cancel the luncheon Friday, and see what you can work out," he said.

I seriously considered applying for the travel promotions job, but did I really want to take an inferior job after so many years at the top, just for the joy of working? If not here, maybe somewhere else.

If I was leaving the job I created so many years ago, at least I would leave on my terms, and I worked out a retirement that was very favorable to me.

But the fact was, I wasn't ready to retire. I loved my job... gathering articles about interesting people and places to visit, sailing on cruise ship inaugurals, crisscrossing the world to collect stories... and 78 didn't seem like the end of the world to me. Still, who would hire a 78-year-old editor?

Ah, but the wonderful thing about being a writer is that you can do it in your own home and no one needs to know your age.

A mantra my mother used to quote to me was: "Man, as the reflection of God, has infinite capabilities, limitless opportunities and ceaseless occupation."

Age played no part in that quotation. I only needed to know that I had infinite intelligence and limitless ideas and the right opportunity would present itself to me.

On the other hand, another favorite family phrase was "God

helps him who helps himself!" I couldn't just sit home and wait for that opportunity to come to me.

I got on the Internet and started looking for writing opportunities.

There were offerings galore, but unfortunately most of them were in New York, and I was firmly situated in Clearwater, Florida. I had enjoyed a long and successful career. Perhaps it was time to sit back and enjoy beach living.

My age was against me, that was for sure. Or was it? Did my years of travel, coupled with my editing experience, count for something? I should not buy into the belief that I had outlived my usefulness. My body was not as mobile as it used to be, but my mind was as active as ever.

I returned to the Internet and started job-hunting again. And there, as if by Divine plan, was an ad for a travel writer in St. Petersburg. Perfect! I could write from home, and the employer never needed to know how old I was.

I dashed off a letter relating how I had ridden camels in Egypt and elephants in India, gone ballooning in France and mountain climbing in Africa and now was ready to freelance as a travel writer.

I didn't have to wait long for an answer. The publisher was interested in my background, would I come to his office for an interview?

My heart sank. I was not a gray-haired old lady with a shawl and a cane, but I was no young chick either. The important thing, I told myself, was to let him see that I had fresh, young ideas and the "go-get-em" spirit to go with them.

I climbed the stairs to his second floor office, strode into the waiting room and announced myself. The publisher was young and attractive, obviously enterprising and surprisingly interested.

For the next hour I laid out my ideas, entertained him with stories of my adventures and prayed that my age didn't stand in the way of freelancing some articles for him.

As I wound up my presentation, he leaned back in his chair, locked his fingers across his chest and was thoughtful. Then he said, "I think you're just the person I'm looking for to be editor of my magazine. Could you start right away?"

As simply as that, I became editor of *Marco Polo* travel magazine, with far-flung trips to exotic places like Mumbai and Dubai and Shanghai and destinations I'd only dreamed of. And all from the comfort of my Florida condo.

And all because I'd realized that ideas are not only limitless, they're also ageless, and your value is as infinite as you allow it to be, so you can find ceaseless occupation.

～ Phyllis W. Zeno ～

Don't Accept Labels

Introduction

My friend has a sister who never did well in school but always had a sharp eye for beauty and artistry. One day my friend was fussing over some flowers in a vase but just couldn't get them to look right. Her sister came along, and with a few deft waves of her hand, transformed them into a stunning bouquet. When praised for having this amazing ability, the sister shrugged off the compliment. She simply didn't view her creative flair as anything special.

Too often we underestimate our own talents in this way. Maybe it's because we've been conditioned to believe that only intellectual abilities like a high I.Q., a gift for mathematics or a large vocabulary have cognitive value. I was fortunate to learn otherwise at a young age.

When I entered high school, a guidance counselor told my mother I wasn't college material because I had performed miserably on the spelling section of a standardized test. Thankfully my mother recognized my other intellectual gifts and stood up for me, insisting I be put into the college-track curriculum. This experience literally defined the course of my life. It showed me how important it is not to accept a label someone else put on me and it allowed me to realize my full potential. Although I still can't spell to save my life it hasn't stopped me from saving the lives of others—or for that matter, from writing a book.

Howard Gardner, Ph.D., a prominent Harvard researcher,

also believes that intelligence isn't limited to a quantifiable I.Q. number or how well you perform in school. In the early 1980's, he pioneered the concept of "multiple intelligences," which is the idea that I.Q. doesn't represent all of the incredible facets and talents of the human brain. In his book, *Frames of Mind: The Theory of Multiple Intelligences*, he suggested that intelligence is not limited to a traditional interpretation but instead encompasses a wide range of cognitive abilities.

According to Gardner, people who have an innate sense of rhythm or an ear for perfect pitch possess a type of intelligence known as musicality. Skilled dancers, gymnasts and ice skaters have an abundance of bodily-kinesthetic intelligence. And my friend's sister, the one with the eye for arranging flowers and making things beautiful? Gardner would say she had keen spatial intelligence, a trait enjoyed by all true artists. As for those who always seem to say the right thing at the right time and are really good at reading people, he refers to that as interpersonal intelligence.

Gardner also hypothesized that traditional I.Q. is not as concrete and unchangeable as some believe. For example, a child who has an easy time learning how to multiply isn't necessarily the class's math whiz. It could be that some children who don't catch onto math right away may benefit from a different teaching approach, one that's better suited to the way their brains work. Others might actually be processing the information on a deeper and more complex level than the speedier student so it takes them a bit longer to put it all together. And of course, it's also entirely possible that some kids will never be good at math and instead possess a brain primed to excel in other areas like writing, piano, woodworking or coaching, areas that might wind up taking them very far in life.

What I love about the multiple intelligences theory is that it allows you to reframe your own abilities and talents, especially those that don't necessarily fit into neat academic boxes. You've probably done some things in your life you sensed were special or even exceptional but dismissed them as no big deal because it wasn't something for which you could receive a grade or diploma. It turns out those outside-the-lines skills have genuine value, which may explain why a high I.Q. doesn't necessarily predict personal success in life.

While it's true one must meet a basic threshold of intelligence for achievement, the analytical skills measured by I.Q. do not tell the whole story. This is why we should celebrate all of our talents and abilities. They're part of what makes your individual brain so wonderful and unique.

The Ordinary Is Really Extraordinary

Most brains are equipped with some basic software that allows us to perform countless functions from the basic to the complex. We know this thanks to innovative technology such as the functional magnetic resonance imaging (fMRI) brain scans that allow us to watch brain activity in real time. Regional changes in blood flow, which are captured on a computer, "light up" under a specific set of circumstances, indicating which areas are performing the task at hand. This window into the workings of the brain allows scientists to "map out" and better understand the brain's extraordinary myriad of capabilities.

Of course there are still infinite mysteries left in the frontiers of neuroscience. For one thing, we don't know how thoughts are generated or how each part of the brain speaks up to ask for additional blood flow or how the brain elects to fulfill these requests. The multitude of everyday skills we usually take for granted are truly remarkable acts of neuro-processing.

Take for instance, *prosody*. Prosody of speech refers to the variances of tone, inflection, pitch, rhythm and loudness in the spoken word that allows the listener to infer meaning that is deeper than the words themselves. Words provide one layer of meaning in conversation. We rely on prosody to convey intent.

Let me give you an example: Let's say your friend says to you, "It's 8 a.m." If his voice is at a higher pitch than usual and he's speaking in an upbeat, happy manner he's probably conveying excitement, perhaps because that means it's time to catch a plane to Aruba. However, if his voice is filled with dread it could be that it's time to head to traffic court. If he ends the statement by lifting up the last word in a questioning tone he may be wondering if it's 8:00 a.m. or not. And if his tone is dripping with sarcasm he may be teasing you about the fact that you have to go to work while he has the day off.

Because of prosody, most of us are capable of catching the true intent of someone's words. What's really incredible — and the part we take most for granted — is that the brain makes these calculations instantaneously and effortlessly.

Not all brains do this so easily. People diagnosed with certain conditions such as autism and some people who've suffered from a brain injury often aren't capable of detecting or imparting prosody. If you say "It's 8 a.m." to someone like this, they have no way of telling whether this fact makes you happy, sad, worried or angry. Conversely, if they say, "It's 8:00 a.m." it may come off as flat and unemotional, whether they are late for an important meeting or awaiting a phone call from a loved one. You can see what a disadvantage this can be. Without the benefit of prosody, the richness, depth and context of the spoken word is lost.

Unusual Tradeoffs

While those with neurological handicaps that are either congenital or acquired may improve prosody and other diminished skills with therapy and hard work, there are other instances where the brain learns to compensate in a novel way. For example, someone born with congenital blindness doesn't let their occipital cortex, the part of the brain that normally translates sight, go to waste. Instead, this valuable patch of neural real estate is appropriated for use by other senses. So that old adage about blind people having superior hearing? It's absolutely true.

Savantism is another interesting case of how the brain sometimes makes tradeoffs that send it down a road less traveled. Savantism is a rare condition typically characterized by impaired mental, emotional and/or social deficits but also by a mysterious and extraordinary talent. Some savants, like Kim Peek, the character portrayed by Dustin Hoffman in *Rain Man*, have a mind-boggling ability to memorize dates and numbers. Although he couldn't care for himself or even button up his shirt, he was able to simultaneously read adjacent pages of a book, one page with one eye and the opposing page with the other eye; and with his photographic memory he was able to retain everything he ever read. Others are math prodigies, musical virtuosos or gifted artists.

There are so few true savants that they aren't well studied. Neuroscientists have only recently begun to focus on what makes their brains so distinctive and currently, there's no consensus about what allows them to do what they do. Whatever makes them tick, it's a testament to the astounding potential of the human mind. I've often wondered if we will ever be able to understand the neural mechanisms that allow them to perform such amazing feats. If so, will it someday help us all perform at a higher level?

Never Set Limits

I find the spectrum of brain abilities fascinating. They demonstrate how ingenious the brain can be. Throughout my career in neurology I've cared for patients with a wide spectrum of neurological conditions and marveled at the brain's ability to overcome and compensate for injury, disease and deficiencies. Those who ultimately do the best are the ones who stay motivated and push themselves to overcome obstacles. It can be frustrating for them to relearn the basics like speaking, reading or holding a utensil, but if they persevere they're usually rewarded. They may not make up all their lost ground but they certainly do better than those who give up. Sometimes they even discover unexpected cognitive treasures along the way by digging deep into their gray matter. For example, a person who has trouble speaking due to stroke may learn to express him or herself through painting or sculpture. In the story "Just a Little Farther to Go" Jan Keller's son John worked hard to restore the skills he lost due to a traumatic brain injury. It can be done.

This is a valuable lesson for us all. Too often it isn't until we or a loved one suffer a catastrophic event that we fully appreciate the magnificence of the human mind. Those challenged with an unfortunate brain event aren't the only ones who benefit from a brain improvement program. Few successful people got to where they are on natural ability alone. They worked hard, practiced, learned, struggled, stayed focused and weathered plenty of setbacks along the way. In the process they were nurturing and structuring their brain for success.

Not all success stories start out with a huge bank account or a superior education either. History is overflowing with individuals who came from humble means and through hard work and unrelenting dedication, went on to achieve great things. Leonardo da Vinci started life as an illegitimate child and grew up an uneducated peasant, yet he made important contributions in every field from art to architecture to astronomy. Oprah Winfrey went from a little girl dressed in a potato sack to one of the most powerful media moguls of all time. Both of these individuals are examples of someone who had natural talent, but more critically, had the drive to hone their innate intellectual aptitude into something exceptional.

Every one of us is capable of achieving something amazing, regardless of circumstance or prior experience. Remember when I told you every brain was unique? I meant it. Once you learn not to set limits on yourself or accept labels, you open yourself up to possibilities you may never have considered before. I sometimes think about what would have happened had I accepted that guidance counselor's assessment of me. Chances are I never would have had the opportunity to attend medical school or for that matter, college. I'm grateful I had enough faith in myself to believe in my capabilities, and the support of parents who encouraged me to pursue my dreams.

Age Is Just a Number

I want to point out one label in particular many people seem willing to accept as a limitation: Age. So often we believe (or we're told) that we're too old to achieve something of value. I'm not saying that you have much chance of winning an Olympic medal if you've reached retirement age, but there's no reason you can't go back to school, write a novel or start a new business once you've celebrated five plus decades of birthdays. It's never too late to try something new or explore undeveloped talents, skills or passions.

If you have goals and dreams but have held yourself back because you think you're too old, think of all the late blooming role models out there who made their mark in the second half of their lives. There's Julia Child, the famous chef who didn't publish her first set of recipes until she was 52; Mahatma Gandhi, the champion of peaceful resistance, who didn't enter politics until well into his fifties; Grandma Moses the celebrated painter, who was in her mid-seventies before she first picked up a paint brush. Oh, and that Olympic medal? Maybe not so impossible after all. Oscar Swahn of Sweden won a gold medal in shooting in the 1912 Olympics at the age of 64 and an Olympic silver medal at the ripe young age of 72.

I think this is one of the reasons I love Phyllis Zeno's "Ageless Occupation" story so much. Forced to attend her own retirement party? Not Phyllis! Instead, at the age of 78, she reinvented herself as a freelance travel writer and continued to challenge her mind. That takes imagination and courage. She's a role model for us all.

Let me also put in a word for the same concept in reverse. Young people can make incredible contributions to the world too. It's true that a teenager isn't eligible to run for president, but teens can surely study hard, get involved in politics and lay the groundwork for future ambitions. I like to think of cognitive capabilities as a work in progress. It's never too early or too late to start building and enriching your brain's cognitive reserve, which you may remember from Chapter 1 is the brain's fund of knowledge and experience. From the moment you are born and throughout your entire life, your cognitive reserve accepts deposits and rewards you with dividends.

Breaking Down Limits

Have you set goals in the past but never followed through because you didn't have the confidence to pursue them? Is there something you have always wanted to do but never quite started? Often this is because we set limits on ourselves. We don't believe we have the required talent or skill. In short, we label ourselves as not being good enough, not having what it takes. If you've held back and haven't tried something because you lacked the education or experience, it's never too late to gain either of these. Your brain never loses its capacity to learn and practice.

You may find it helpful to take an inventory of your strengths, even if up until now you've felt they're trivial. My friend's sister may not consider her ability to rearrange flowers as anything special, but a good sense of style and beauty is a considerable asset in many careers and aspects of life. As Gardner points out, this is a form of intelligence in its own right. You probably have talents and abilities like this that up until now may have seemed insignificant. It's also possible that these skills lay dormant because they were never properly nurtured in the most optimal learning environment for you personally.

If for example, your cerebral gifts are in the realm of kinesthetics, it's likely that you learn best by moving and doing, while someone who is more linguistically endowed will learn best through lectures and listening. So take some time to consider your true strengths, and with a little thought, training and practice one of these talents might be put to good use and flourish.

Age aside, I also do love the idea of "cognitive role models." At Harvard I'm surrounded by some of the best and brightest minds in the medical world. While it's easy to be intimidated by their sheer brilliance, I remind myself to focus on how incredibly fortunate I am to have so many fascinating and accomplished people to learn from. Every day, they inspire me to think in new ways and strive to improve.

You probably know a few people who use their minds in a way you admire and wish to emulate. Try to spend more time with these people so you can understand how they've modeled their brains for achievement. Even if you may only know some of your role models from the pages of a magazine or a history book, read everything you can about them. Find out how they spend their time, their habits, and how they live their lives. In the process, you will discover the key to how they nurtured and groomed their brains for success. By applying the same methods, you too can maximize your own mental faculties and ultimately realize your full potential.

The Multiple Intelligences

Gardner believed that the concept of intelligence applies to more than just how well you perform on an IQ test. Do you see your innate talents somewhere on this list? Are you surprised to learn that something you do well might be considered a type of intelligence?

Linguistic intelligence involves sensitivity to spoken and written language, the ability to learn languages, and the capacity to use language to accomplish certain goals.

Logical-mathematical intelligence consists of the capacity to analyze problems logically, carry out mathematical operations, and investigate issues scientifically.

Musical intelligence encompasses skill in the performance, composition, and appreciation of musical patterns, sounds, rhythms and tones.

Bodily-kinesthetic intelligence includes hand-eye coordination, handling objects skillfully and control of body movement.

Spatial intelligence deals with spatial judgment and the ability to visualize with the mind's eye.

Interpersonal intelligence is concerned with the capacity to understand the intentions, motivations, moods and desires of other people.

Intrapersonal intelligence entails the capacity to understand yourself and to appreciate your own feelings, motivations and actions.

Naturalistic intelligence refers to being in tune with nature and an aptitude for understanding natural surroundings, including animals, plants and landscapes.

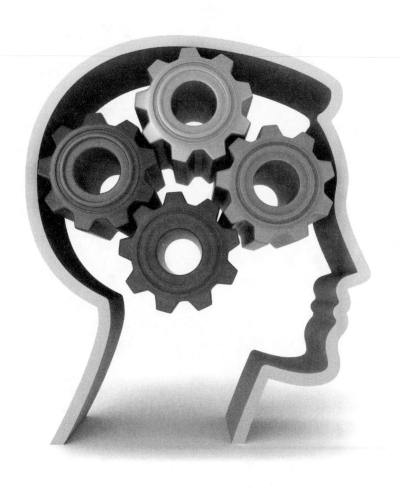

Meet Our Contributors
Meet the Authors
Acknowledgments

Meet Our Contributors

Debbie Acklin currently focuses her writing on nonfiction short stories, but plans on trying her hand at fiction very soon. She loves to travel and read (of course). She may be contacted at her website www.debbieacklin.com.

Teresa Ambord writes business articles from her home in rural northern California. She also writes about her family and her pets. Teresa is fully owned by her dogs that inspire her writing and decorate her life. She volunteers as a foster parent for animals, at ACAWL.org. E-mail her at ambertrees@charter.net.

Garrett Bauman and his wife live in upstate New York's Finger Lakes region. He has challenged several raccoons to toss handkerchiefs with him, but all have declined. After a career teaching at Monroe Community College, he now writes for many magazines and revises his college textbooks. E-mail him at mbauman@retiree.monroecc.edu.

Anna (Betty) Brack is an 87-year-old woman who was given a great gift at birth—a curious brain. She knows how blessed she has been to have had such an interesting life filled with family, friends, work and travel. She fills her time with reading, e-mail, web surfing and now, a new hobby, writing!

Christine Catlin is a high school student in Minnesota. When not writing she enjoys playing sports, reading, and learning new things!

Beth Cato resides in Arizona with her husband and son. She's an associate member of the Science Fiction & Fantasy Writers of America, with stories in various anthologies and magazines. This is her sixth time published in a *Chicken Soup for the Soul* book. For information on her latest projects, please visit www.bethcato.com.

Stephanie Davenport is a wife, mom and pastor. She was previously a columnist and correspondent for the *Mahomet Citizen*. Her writing has been published in *Chicken Soup for the Soul: Food and Love*, Christianity Today's *Marriage Partnership*, *Discipleship Journal*, *Cutting Edge* and *Focus on the Family*. She blogs at stephaniedavenport.wordpress.com.

Shawnelle Eliasen and her husband Lonny raise their five sons in Illinois. Shawnelle home teaches her youngest boys. Her writing has been published in *Guideposts*, *MomSense* magazine, *Marriage Partnership*, *A Cup of Comfort* books, numerous *Chicken Soup for the Soul* books, and other anthologies. Follow her adventures at Shawnellewrites.blogspot.com.

Patricia Gordon holds degrees in music education from Illinois State University and Western Michigan University. A retired elementary teacher, she now teaches at Grand Valley State University. Patty enjoys traveling and crafting — sewing, crocheting, and scrapbooking are current favorites. She writes fiction as Patricia Kiyono. Learn more at patriciakiyono.com.

Kim Hackett lives in Tampa Bay with her husband and two children. She taught kindergarten for 15 years, and now enjoys her time as a stay-at-home mom. She's had several short stories published and is currently putting the final touches on her first novel. E-mail her at khackett@tampabay.rr.com.

Cathy C. Hall is a writer from Georgia. Her published works include essays, stories, poems and articles for both children and adults. And she manages to work in a contest or two as well! Find out if she wins at cathychall.wordpress.com.

Jennie Ivey lives in Tennessee. She is the author of numerous fiction and nonfiction works, including stories in several *Chicken Soup for the Soul* anthologies. Her latest book is *Soldiers, Spies & Spartans: Civil War Stories from Tennessee*. Visit her website at www.jennieivey.com.

Jan Keller graduated from Baylor College of Dentistry as a dental hygienist. She is an ordained minister with Global Spheres, Inc. in Denton, TX. Jan currently lives in South Texas with James, her husband of 41 years. Together they have four children and 11 grandchildren.

Eve Legato graduated from Hampshire College in 2007 and has since held several positions in the publishing industry. She is a frequent contributor to the *Chicken Soup for the Soul* series.

Simon Lewis is a film and television producer. Simon's the author of *Rise and Shine: The Extraordinary Story of One Man's Journey from Near Death to Full Recovery*, which uses his experiences to explore consciousness and recovery. Simon plans to write further inspirational books and presentations. Please visit www.riseandshinethebook.com and e-mail Simon at zermatt1@gmail.com.

Stephen D. Rogers (www.stephendrogers.com) is the editor of *My First Year in the Classroom*, the author of *A Dictionary of Made-Up Languages*, and a contributor to hundreds of publications including the following *Chicken Soup for the Soul* titles: *Empty Nesters, Grandma's, Mother of Preschooler's,* and *Thanks Mom.*

Diana Savage, the principal at Savage Creative Services, LLC, has a master's degree in theological studies. Although her ability with numbers is improving, she still prefers working with words as a writer, editor, and public speaker. She also loves reading books to her grandson. Diana can be reached via e-mail at info@DianaSavage.com.

John Scanlan is a 1983 graduate of the United States Naval Academy, and retired from the Marine Corps as a Lieutenant Colonel aviator. He currently resides on Hilton Head Island, SC, and is pursuing a second career as a writer. John can be reached via e-mail at ping1@hargray.com.

Lindy Schneider is an author, illustrator, playwright and speaker but NOT an improv actor! Her plays have been performed on various stages throughout Phoenix and she is currently working on a movie script. Contact her at lindy_schn@yahoo.com or www.LindysBooks.com.

Jacqueline Seewald taught high school English and also creative, expository and technical writing at Rutgers University. She's worked as an academic librarian and an educational media specialist. Eleven of her books have been published. Her short stories, poems, essays, reviews and articles have appeared in hundreds of magazines, newspapers and anthologies.

Annmarie B. Tait resides in Conshohocken, PA, with her husband Joe Beck. In addition to writing stories, Annmarie enjoys cooking, crocheting and singing. Annmarie has stories published in several *Chicken Soup for the Soul* volumes and has also been nominated for a 2012 Pushcart Literary Award. E-mail Annmarie at irishbloom@aol.com.

Marla H. Thurman lives in Signal Mountain, TN, with her dogs Jasper and Sophie. She is currently working on a memoir. Her dream is that one day her favorite author, Pat Conroy, will ask for her autograph.

L.D. Whitaker attended a two-room school in the Ozarks and survived the sixties and the University of Missouri School of Law. His debut novel, *Geese to a Poor Market*, won the Ozark Writer's League Best Book of the Year Award. He lives with his wife and two standard poodles in rural Missouri. E-mail him at info@geesetoapoormarket.com.

Pat Williams is the senior vice president of the NBA's Orlando Magic. Also a popular corporate speaker, Pat has authored over 75 books, including *Chicken Soup for the Soul: Inside Basketball*. Contact Pat via his website at www.patWilliamsMotivate.com.

Dallas Woodburn is the author of two collections of short stories and editor of *Dancing With The Pen: a collection of today's best youth writing*. Her essays and fiction have appeared in numerous publications including *Family Circle*, *Los Angeles Times*, and *Writer's Digest*. Learn more at www.writeonbooks.org and http://dallaswoodburn.blogspot.com.

Phyllis W. Zeno was the founding editor of AAA *Going Places* for 29 years. When she retired in 2004, she became publisher/editor of *Marco Polo* magazine. She is now a freelance writer for *Cruise Travel* and has been published in eight *Chicken Soup for the Soul* books.

Meet Our Authors

Marie Pasinski, MD graduated from Harvard Medical School where she continues to serve on the faculty. She is a board certified member of the American Academy of Neurology and a staff neurologist at Massachusetts General Hospital. Dr. Pasinski cares for patients with a broad range of neurologic disorders. Her special interests include brain health, dementia prevention and the effects of mental stimulation, exercise, diet, and socialization, on the brain. By optimizing the brain's remarkable ability to redesign itself through her seven-step program, Dr. Pasinski believes that a healthier, more vibrant brain can be achieved at any age.

Dr. Pasinski has been featured as an expert commentator for the *Today* show, *Ladies' Home Journal*, *Woman's World* magazine and numerous other media outlets. She is a frequent guest speaker at conferences and symposia, writes a health column for The Huffington Post and is the author of *Beautiful Brain, Beautiful You*.

A renowned brain expert, Dr. Pasinski is dedicated to increasing public awareness about the importance of adopting a brain healthy lifestyle and the realization that our brains are the true source of our vitality and happiness. Dr. Pasinski practices what she teaches: at age 40 she started taking piano lessons for the first time and more recently she has been honing her writing skills, studying improv and competing in triathlons. She lives in Massachusetts with her husband and has raised two sons.

To learn more, please visit her interactive website at www.MariePasinski.com.

Liz Neporent is a health, fitness and medical writer who has written more than 15 books including the bestsellers *The Winner's Brain: 8 Strategies Great Minds Use to Achieve Success* and *Weight Training for Dummies*. She is a regular contributor to dozens of websites, publications and national media outlets. She is on the emeritus board of directors and a national spokesperson for the American Council on Exercise and the fitness and social media advisor for The Hudson Valley Women's Health Initiative, a charitable organization dedicated to educating people about medical issues, health and fitness. She lives in New York City with her husband Jay and daughter Skylar. Follow her on twitter @lizzyfit or check out her website www.liznep.com.

Acknowledgments

My gratitude to all the contributing writers for sharing their inspirational stories. I hope to have the opportunity to meet each of you someday. Special thanks to Anna (Betty) Brack for the wisdom and many stories you have shared with me including the one you wrote for this book.

I'd like to offer some very special thank yous. To Amy Newmark, my publisher at Chicken Soup for the Soul — your creative guidance, expertise and availability throughout this project have been exceptional. It was truly a pleasure to work with you. And to Dr. Julie Silver of Harvard Health Publications — when I first took your writing course, publishing a book was a dream and here we are on number two! These two outstanding women made this book a reality. Thank you for making my dreams come true.

To Liz Neporent — my writer and brainstorming partner. Who knew writing a book could be so much fun? I so enjoyed collaborating with you. Your wonderful sense of humor and brilliance come from a most beautiful brain!

I am forever grateful to the women who nurture my mind and my soul. To my dear friend and gifted artist, Karin Stanley, you are an artist in every sense of the word, discovering and encouraging the talents of those who are lucky enough to count you as a friend. To the Goddesses in my life: Diane Dunfee, Rebecca Flacke, Mary Flannery, Patty Forster, Ute Gfrerer, Linda Hall, Christine Kendall, Cora Long, Louise Rusk, and Suzanne Tarlov. Thank you for the intimate conversations and countless laughs we share on our "facial nights" which rejuvenate my life as well as my complexion! My heartfelt thanks to Linda Hall (Goddess of Kindness) for your thoughtful comments on the manuscript — I cherish your friendship. And to Linda Leum, Lorinda de Zayas, Perla Thulin and Patricia Dabbah — though separated by distance, you are close at heart.

With deep appreciation to all the brilliant minds at Harvard I'm so fortunate to know, especially Drs. Shahram Khoshbin, Misha Pless and Herbert Benson. Thanks to Rusty Shelton, Amber McGinty and Beth Gwazdosky at Shelton Interactive for all that you do. To Sheena (Nancy) Sarles, Mary Valentine King, Sheila Arsenault, Deb Mahoney, Lil Carter and Duke Bradley — for always being there. And to John Mottern — photographer extraordinaire!

To my parents, Richard and Patricia Burke, you always encouraged me to discover my true potential and reach for the stars. For that and your unending love and support, I will always be grateful. To my brothers Rich, Mike and Jude Burke — I'm the luckiest sister in the world because of you.

To my sons Eric and Stephen, I treasure our time together and admire the young men you have become. Most of all, my deepest gratitude to my husband Roger. The publication date of this book marks the anniversary of that first evening you walked into the Budapest Restaurant and I served you up some Hungarian delicacies. I was captivated by your kindness, integrity and humor.... some things never change. Thank you Roger for 30 wonderful years.

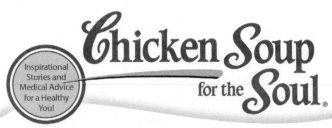

Chicken Soup for the Soul.

Inspirational Stories and Medical Advice for a Healthy You!

by **DR. JEFF BROWN** of
HARVARD MEDICAL SCHOOL
with **LIZ NEPORENT**

Say Goodbye to Stress

Manage Your Problems, Big and Small, Every Day

Fantastic advice on how to reduce stress and restore serenity to your life. Who knew it could be so easy?
~ Dr. Amy Gagliardi

Chicken Soup for the Soul:
Say Goodbye to Stress
978-1-935096-88-7
ebook: 978-1-611592-09-2

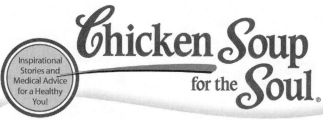

Chicken Soup for the Soul.

Inspirational
Stories and
Medical Advice
for a Healthy
You!

by DR. SUZANNE KOVEN of HARVARD MEDICAL SCHOOL

Say Hello to a Better Body!

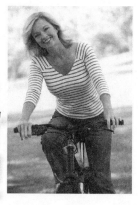

Weight Loss and Fitness for Women Over 50

A great combination of intelligent advice and
inspirational stories—women over 50 *can* look
and feel fabulous! ~ Dr. Elizabeth Pegg Frates

Chicken Soup for the Soul:
Say Hello to a Better Body!
978-1-935096-89-4
ebook: 978-1-611592-12-2

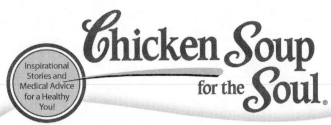

Chicken Soup for the Soul

Inspirational Stories and Medical Advice for a Healthy You!

for the Soul®

by **DR. JULIE SILVER** of
HARVARD MEDICAL SCHOOL

Say Goodbye to Back Pain!

How to Handle Flare-Ups, Injuries, and Everyday Back Health

Terrific tips for flare-ups *and* for chronic back pain.
You'll be back in action sooner than you think!
~ Dr. Howard Ezra Lewine

Chicken Soup for the Soul:
Say Goodbye to Back Pain!
978-1-935096-87-0
ebook: 978-1-611592-08-5

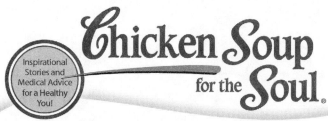

Chicken Soup for the Soul

for the Soul

Inspirational Stories and Medical Advice for a Healthy You!

by DR. JEFF BROWN of
HARVARD MEDICAL SCHOOL

Think Positive
for
Great
Health

Use Your Mind to Promote Your Own Healing and Wellness

Solid advice and transformative stories —
a true path to a positive outlook and great health!
~ Dr. Arthur J. Siegel

Chicken Soup for the Soul:
Think Positive for Great Health
978-1-935096-90-0
ebook: 978-1-611592-13-9

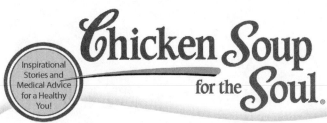

Inspirational Stories and Medical Advice for a Healthy You!

Chicken Soup for the Soul.

by **DR. JULIE SILVER** of
HARVARD MEDICAL SCHOOL

Hope & Healing for Your Breast Cancer Journey

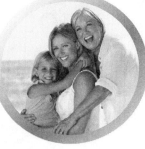

Surviving and Thriving During and After Your Diagnosis and Treatment

Every woman diagnosed with breast cancer deserves excellent emotional and medical support—this book delivers both! ~Dr. Kimberly Allison

Chicken Soup for the Soul:
Hope & Healing for Your Breast Cancer Journey
978-1-935096-94-8
ebook: 978-1-611592-11-5